Palgrave Studies in Public Health Policy Research

Series Editors
Patrick Fafard, Global Strategy Lab, University of Ottawa, Ottawa, ON, Canada
Evelyne de Leeuw, Liverpool Hospital, CHETRE, University of New South Wales, Liverpool, NSW, Australia

Public health has increasingly cast the net wider. The field has moved on from a hygiene perspective and infectious and occupational disease base (where it was born in the 19th century) to a concern for unhealthy lifestyles post-WWII, and more recently to the uneven distribution of health and its (re)sources. It is of course interesting that these 'paradigms' in many places around the world live right next to each other. Hygiene, lifestyles, and health equity form the complex (indeed, wicked) policy agendas for health and social/sustainable development. All of these, it is now recognized, are part of the 'social determinants of health'.

The broad new public health agenda, with its multitude of competing issues, professions, and perspectives requires a much more sophisticated understanding of government and the policy process. In effect, there is a growing recognition of the extent to which the public health community writ large needs to better understand government and move beyond what has traditionally been a certain naiveté about politics and the process of policy making. Public health scholars and practitioners have embraced this need to understand, and influence, how governments at all levels make policy choices and decisions. Political scientists and international relations scholars and practitioners are engaging in the growing public health agenda as it forms an interesting expanse of glocal policy development and implementation.

Broader, more detailed, and more profound scholarship is required at the interface between health and political science. This series will thus be a powerful tool to build bridges between political science, international relations and public health. It will showcase the potential of rigorous political and international relations science for better understanding public health issues. It will also support the public health professional with a new theoretical and methodological toolbox. The series will include monographs (both conventional and shorter Pivots) and collections that appeal to three audiences: scholars of public health, public health practitioners, and members of the political science community with an interest in public health policy and politics.

Patrick Harris

Illuminating Policy for Health

Insights From a Decade of Researching Urban and Regional Planning

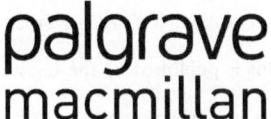

Patrick Harris
Centre for Health Equity Training
Research and Evaluation, Centre
for Primary Health Care and Equity
University of New South Wales
Sydney, NSW, Australia

This work was supported by the Australian Research Council, the Australian National Health and Medical Research Council, the Henry Halloran Trust at Sydney University, and the Balnaves Foundation at Sydney University.

Palgrave Studies in Public Health Policy Research
ISBN 978-3-031-13198-1   ISBN 978-3-031-13199-8   (eBook)
https://doi.org/10.1007/978-3-031-13199-8

Cover image: © MELBA PHOTO AGENCY/Alamy Stock Photo

This Palgrave Macmillan imprint is published by the registered company Springer Nature Switzerland AG
The registered company address is: Gewerbestrasse 11, 6330 Cham, Switzerland

I'd like to dedicate this book to my wife, Dan, and kids, Charlie and Finn. Yes, boys, I am a real Doctor, just one that does research.

ACKNOWLEDGEMENTS

I have many people to acknowledge here, and I hope I mention all of those who have helped me over the years.

I would especially like to mention Peter Sainsbury, my Ph.D. supervisor who became a colleague and friend both scholastically and editorially over the last decade. I hope I have found my voice, Peter.

Other special mention goes to Evelyne De Leeuw. So much support over such a long time, so thanks from the bottom of my heart. Onward now together to so many exciting opportunities!

Sharon Friel and Fran Baum for ongoing intellectual collaborations (and friendships). Respective teams ditto (Ashley Schram, Bel Townsend, Toby Freeman, Matt Fisher, Anna Zeirch and Tamara MacKean). Dennis McDermott was a vital influence and colleague and is sadly missed.

Liz and Mark Harris get stand-alone mention for giving me my first job and then sticking with me across the rest of it.

Andrew Wilson for all the mentoring support over much of the life of the research reported here. The team at Menzies Centre for Health Policy for putting up with me, including pragmatic advice from Steve Leeder and Penny Hawe. And finally, Anne-Marie Thow for being my public policy and health partner in crime. I enjoyed my time with you all.

Thanks finally to the two reviewers whose suggestions strengthened the manuscript enormously.

Funding

A raft of different funders and fundings sources supported the research. The National Health and Medical Research Council funded my early career fellowship and our Centre for Research Excellence that directly informed the research. The Australian Research Council funded additional aspects to the research, especially our cross case comparative work with South Australia.

The Henry Halloran Trust at Sydney University provided additional funds for the case studies Environmental Assessment and Sydney Focussed Strategic Planning case studies. The Balnaves Foundation at Sydney University funded the infrastructure focussed aspect of the research.

Sydney University also supported me with a bridging funding which helped provide the space to complete the research.

Since then, my dual role at the University of New South Wales and South Western Sydney Local Health District has provided a wonderful home from which to complete the writing of the book (and to progress working on some of the recommendations!).

Praise for *Illuminating Policy for Health*

"Harris has extensive experience in public health policy research, and he uses it to great effect in this book. His aim is to use what we know about public health problems, and policy processes, to inform sophisticated policy analysis. This approach requires analysts to situate their potential policy solutions in the context of a political audience more or less receptive to their ideas, and a complex policymaking environment out of their full understanding and control."

—Paul Cairney, *Professor of Politics and Public Policy, University of Stirling, UK*

"Turning the floodlights on healthy public policy, Patrick Harris adopts a Critical Realist lens to highlight the importance of theory, framing, policy and governance in metropolitan planning, urban transport infrastructure, impact assessment, coal mining and climate change. Supported by raw and insightful observations about his personal navigation of research and writing, *Illuminating Policy for Health* is a must-read for anybody interested in the nexus of urban and regional planning and health policy."

—Phil McManus, *Professor of Urban and Environmental Geography, The University of Sydney, Australia*

"This book applies a critical lens to understanding policy from a public health perspective. Using urban governance as a case study (a policy area in much need of greater public health attention, given the current climate emergency), Harris demonstrates the fundamentally political nature of policymaking. It should be of interest to anyone interested in better understanding the ways politics and power shape policy outcomes."

—Katherine Smith, *Professor of Health Policy, University of Strathclyde, UK*

CONTENTS

LIST OF FIGURES

LIST OF TABLES

CHAPTER 1

Introduction

This book stems from over a decade of work to better understand 'healthy public policy'. 'Healthy public policy' and derivatives like 'health in all policies' speak to the vast evidence base linking public policy with people's health. The architects of public health in the nineteenth century were driven by the understanding that people living and employed in cramped and unsanitary conditions faced devastating risks to their health. Fast forward to today and this proposition remains very real. COVID-19 is the most famous recent example; a virus first experienced in a wet-market in a highly urbanised area of China essentially morphed into a pandemic which shut the world down. Climate change is another. Energy, food and transport demands, mostly from cities, have stretched the climate to the extent that human health is constantly and increasingly at risk from the changes that have been wrought. Public policy decisions drive these health impacts and their uneven and inequitable spread in the population. Ergo, a fundamental task is influencing public policy to be 'healthy'.

The Palgrave series this book belongs intends to provide a body of work that articulates the connections between public health and public policy. I was invited to write this book because that is what my work does. In terms of topics, the book touches on many of the fundamental policy issues facing public health today: urbanisation, transport, energy, economics and sustainability. I hope the book informs the growing body

P. Harris, *Illuminating Policy for Health*, Palgrave Studies in Public Health Policy Research,
https://doi.org/10.1007/978-3-031-13199-8_1

of people who are professionally interested in the intersection between disciplines. My intent is to present a coherent argument about how public policy works from the perspective of public health. The book, therefore, breaks down public policy into its constituent parts so that I and others can understand and better influence policymaking.

If that idea whets your appetite, read on.

Throughout the book are several overlapping points of focus. The principal aim is to guide policy analysis to understand and influence 'healthy public policy'. The book provides a methodology for sophisticated health focussed policy analysis which situates public health within complex political processes and systems. As I go on to show, public health, when situated in this way, is an idea and a set of values or interests. Those values are accepted or resisted by people who are living and working under institutional rules and mandates. Those rules and mandates, while often implicit, govern those people working to make or influence policy. Those people in turn can influence those rules.

This book is fundamentally about researching public health policy in all its complexity. Part I explains how doing and thinking about research necessarily intertwine in the type of policy analysis the book advocates. Part II applies that methodology in my research investigating how health issues were included in urban and regional planning in New South Wales (and South Australia), Australia.

As a research treatise, the book has a single methodological premise, to develop knowledge about what public health policy is, how it is made and under what conditions. Understanding and explaining what has come to be known as healthy public policy (Harris & Wise, 2020) requires accepting policy as complex but made up of a consistent set of essential characteristics. These characteristics are isolated and explained as the fundamental triggers in systems through which to influence public policy to be 'healthy'. The book offers a methodology that allows policy analysis to develop a coherent explanation of the interconnections between complex forces that result in policy choices and decisions. Typically, the traditional public health research enterprise looks to produce knowledge *for* policy rather than knowledge *about* policymaking. This book's focus is the latter.

In my core discipline of public health, how to go about this type of policy analysis is, I believe, missing from the literature linking health and public policy. 'How to go about' analysing public health policy, or as I refer to it healthy public policy, is an important distinction that sets this book apart from others. This is especially critical in my core discipline, public health, which tends to take a pragmatic approach to research and evidence generation. Public health research *about* policymaking is under-recognised and restricted to the few of us who practise in the dark arts of the social sciences. Limited understanding of what healthy public policy is and how to go about understanding it is a mistake on many levels. Addressing that knowledge gap is the back story to this book.

The 'meta-methodology' which I base the book in, critical realism, helps articulate the goal and strategies to work through healthy public policy's complexities. I (re)introduce and apply the core research and analytic tasks set by critical realism. In doing so, I hope to add an interesting voice, and an important methodology, for others to take up in their pursuit of healthy public policy.

At the outset, it is important to disappoint strident adherents to the critical realist paradigm. I do not intend to emulate Roy Bhaskar, Andrew Sayer and Margaret Archer. Nor do I plan to take on the realist evaluation gurus like Ray Pawson. Rather, I use kernels of their thinking to develop healthy public policy analysis. A dogmatic approach to critical realism as a separate world of knowledge generation is not useful. Worse still, adhering to critical realism tooth and nail is a stylistic nightmare for both writer and reader. Rather, I present to the best of my ability my own narrative while sticking to the fundamental tenets. Sometimes the concepts mean that dense writing is necessary. Overall, I try to avoid that. Or at least warn when it is coming.

I must make a quick introductory point about 'health' from an evidentiary position. The backdrop to this book is my professional and academic immersion into how health and health equity intersect with public policy. As I show in Chapter 2, the evidence base behind taking action to influence healthy public policy is massive. The findings of the World Health Organisation Commission on the Social Determinants of Health, to take but one example, demonstrated the sheer breadth of knowledge about why health inequities are a 'toxic combination of bad policies, economics, and politics' (2009, p. 26). Fast forward to 2021, the same toxic combination is playing out with massive consequences for health and equity: global spread of disease, trans-boundary environmental pollution, burgeoning urban (and slum) populations and increasing health disparities mirroring widening class inequalities (Corburn, 2017). However, in its quest to demonstrate the evidence the WHO Commission did not sufficiently interrogate what policy is. Sure, there was a clear proposition from all the evidence that 'power, resources and money' were at the core of the toxic combination. But interrogating policymaking and politics was overlooked.

Often forgotten in the search for evidence about a problem is the task of understanding what the fundamentals or essentials of that problem are. This challenge is what the critical realist Andrew Sayer sets as 'better conceptualisation of the objects of interest'. I present how to go about this conceptualisation of the object of public health policy in Chapters 2 and 3. The essence of healthy public policy is, of course, public policy. Breaking down public policy into essential parts necessarily follows. That work involves digesting a whole body of knowledge and theory from which to then better conceptualise first what public policy is. For this book, theories about governance, institutions, process, power and politics come into play. I use insights from these theories to explain data about [the object of] healthy urban and regional planning.

There is a strong 'urban' flavour throughout the book. The urban dimension comes about mainly because my research topic of focus, detailed in Part II, was urban and regional planning. The book is aimed at providing the emerging field of 'healthy urban planning' with a detailed account of doing research about healthy urban and regional policy. Many of those working in urban studies or planning have for a long time been thinking and applying about similar themes. Healthy urban planning, as I go on to show, has similar disciplinary orientations to the overarching discipline of public health—that is, developing evidence for healthy urban policy. This book adds to the body of knowledge of research about healthy urban policy.

The overall task is necessarily inter-disciplinary. I owe enormous debt to many methodologists from across the social sciences, especially political science and urban politics, whose contribution shall become clear throughout. That said, up front I also want to pre-empt potential disappointment with my use of theory. A good analogy for the challenge of theoretical navigation is navigating a library collection. There is so much existing knowledge and information that can be brought to bear on public health policy that it is impossible to include everything the library has to offer. I have, as you will come to see, walked through the library with the sole purpose of explaining the complexities of influencing 'healthy public policy' in urban and regional planning. I could not have, and did not want to, digest the whole library. I chose books and the ideas they offer to focus my methodology and then to explain the data that I had collected. My systematic, purposive, use of theory is core to the type of analysis I present; in many ways, this book demonstrates how to use and apply theory as part of a comprehensive analysis of public health policy.

Part I of the book presents the core methodological concepts, premises and ideas behind doing policy analysis in the manner I suggest. I begin with making the connections between health and public policy, with a particular focus on the intersections between health and 'urban' issues. I then set the methodology in critical realism with a peppering of how urban studies and political science can overlap with that methodology. I then drill into that analysis as a method that mixes empirical data with theoretical insights to arrive at deeper, better explanations of how 'healthy' public policy decisions come about.

Part II applies the methodology of Part I. I demonstrate how I systematically applied each aspect of the methodology to my investigation of an urban and regional planning system in New South Wales, Australia. I first break down the essentials of that policy system from the data I collected. I then navigate the various theories of relevance to that data. I then provide a full explanation of that system and how health came to be included or not at various point, and why. I also offer a normative critique of what is necessary to position health into that system, given the findings.

References

Corburn, J. (2017). Equitable and healthy city planning: Towards healthy urban governance in the century of the city. In *Healthy cities* (pp. 31–41). Springer.

Harris, P., & Wise, M. (2020). *Healthy public policy*. Oxford University Press.

Howlett, M., Ramesh, M., & Perl, A. (2009). *Studying public policy: Policy cycles and policy sub-systems* (3rd ed.). Oxford University Press.

PART I

Methodology Matters

Part 1 of the book covers background and methodology, and concludes with an analytic framework. The audience is for those with a broad interest in public health policy. I have retained an urban focus, although that lens really comes into its own in Part II. Here, I focus on public health policy and how to 'illuminate' this with research. I focus first on the history of public health policy. I then switch lanes into critical realist methodology, in Chapter 3, and a roadmap for doing that analysis in Chapter 4. Chapter 5 shifts again, introducing a policy focussed framework that provides the fundamentals for public health policy analysis.

CHAPTER 2

The Positioning of Health in Public Policy (with an Urban Flavour)

Anyone who has attended a cross-sectoral meeting will, at some point before, during or after that encounter, have questioned or been questioned about why they are there. 'What has this encounter got to do with my day-to-day work?' for example, or, if more glass half full, 'what can we achieve together?'. This chapter provides answers to such questions by introducing the history of 'healthy public policy'. In a nutshell, there is a long historical and social premise for including and considering health as a core public policy concern. Importantly, what emerges across the bodies of work reviewed over the chapter is a normative—or 'what ought to be'—focus: public policy ought to positively impact on health equity. This health equity framing as the goal for healthy public policy is the focal point for the work.

It is also worth setting out my view at this point that the premise behind healthy public policy covers the best of what public health[1] has to offer society: a combination of strong empirical evidence with a normative determination to take action to shift policy to benefit human health and wellbeing. This is of course a difficult task. Taking on that challenge is an objective of this book.

---

[1] For those interested in why a supposed neutral position about public health is self-defeating, see https://www.theatlantic.com/health/archive/2021/10/how-public-health-took-part-its-own-downfall/620457/.

© The Author(s), under exclusive license to Springer Nature
Switzerland AG 2022
P. Harris, *Illuminating Policy for Health*, Palgrave Studies
in Public Health Policy Research,
https://doi.org/10.1007/978-3-031-13199-8_2

The purpose of this chapter is also to orient readers to a persistent interest in public health policy over a decent chunk of history. Running throughout the chapter is a tension between technical and strategic approaches. By and large, I argue, the history of public health policy shows that both technical ability and strategic acumen are required. I end the chapter by situating this book as a treatise about how to engage, with a public health focus, in research and analysis 'of policy'.

I also use the chapter to focus on what 'urban' means from a health focussed policy perspective. Living in urbanised environments has historically provided the background for much of why public health policy matters.

Getting language right is important for research and practice (Williams, 2003). 'Framing' ideas is essential to be effective at influencing policy (Rein & Schön, 1994). For example, how 'health' policy ideas are valued and presented has been shown to be crucial for the types of policies that are then developed and implemented with varying influences on health (Smith, 2013). Precision in language and discourse influences the processes that shape policy (Stone, 1997). Discourse provides the boundaries for which type of actors, or policy players, can enter policy discussions or become part of various policy networks (Howarth, 2010; Laumann & Knoke, 1987, Sabatier, 1988). Indeed, the healthy public policy analysis presented in this book is largely about ideas and discourse (Arts & Van Tatenhove, 2004; Carstensen & Schmidt, 2016; Schmidt, 2008).

The presentation of the body of work and action to influence public health policy has morphed over the years in name, but the substance has remained. That body of work is conspicuous in its disciplinary base within public health broadly, and what public health people call 'health promotion' in particular. Retaining the overall title 'Healthy Public Policy' makes sense to me because public policy remains the object of interest. Other ways of framing action to influence public policy for health include 'intersectoral action', 'health in all policies' and most recently 'planetary health'. Of particular interest to urbanists is the 'healthy cities' movement that has had almost as long a life as healthy public policy, and still flourishes (in pockets) today.

Careless use of 'health policy' terminology is problematic for healthy public policy (De Leeuw & Harris, 2022). When 'health policy' is evoked, this by and large means 'public policy for health care'. The outcome of interest tends to be the provision of health services or hospitals or specific diseases. Importantly, especially for this book, a healthcare focus is not the same as healthy public policy. Healthy public policy looks the other way, at *the policies that create a healthy society or those that do not*.

What, then, is healthy public policy?

HEALTHY PUBLIC POLICY: A HISTORY

Healthy public policy (HPP) 'emerged' as an idea for public health in the 1980s, cemented globally by the WHO's Ottawa Charter for Health Promotion. Prior to the Charter, the concept was originally coined by several thinkers and activists including Trevor Hancock—who notably also was a pioneer of healthy cities (Hancock, 1985). Around that time, Nancy Milio wrote her book *Promoting Health through Public Policy* and subsequent excellent introductory articles (Milio, 1981, 1987, 2001). Some of the language is out of date—'ecological' for instance has been replaced by complex systems/network governance—but the core concepts laid down remain relevant today.

Milio (1987), for instance, explains that progress on healthy public policy requires being both 'substantive' and 'strategic'. *Substantive* covers the technical evidence and tools that public health and other disciplines tend to focus research on—generating evidence of the effects of policy options on health impacts or outcomes. *Strategic* is necessarily broader and process oriented, predicated on understanding how options are made 'under various conditions...the best way to find such policy relevant information is by observing and analysing the real-world experience of public policy making' (p. 265).

Public health as a discipline faces a similar dilemma. One the one hand, public health is often thought to be about providing the best technically proficient evidence about the health of the public. COVID-19 is the latest in a long line of societal challenges that has demonstrated the importance of that technical knowledge. But alongside has been a history of public health as being political, requiring tactics and strategies as well as the best available evidence. COVID-19 has repeated the historical embeddedness of health inequalities, laying bare, once again, the need for a strategic public health policy response (Bambra et al., 2021). Heathy public policy (herein HPP) has always been concerned with politics and is in many ways the vanguard of public health's necessary engagement with public policy and politics (Bambra et al., 2005).

An early collection of viewpoints about HPP (Tesh et al., 1987) helps articulate these core political dimensions. Crucially, these viewpoints converged around the need for public policy to impact positively, rather than negatively, on the overall health of the community and its equitable distribution in society—i.e. that good health is shared across the community rather than being associated with socio-economic status (Dahlgren, 1991). The writing is full of gems foundational to understanding the politics in public health policy, including some cautionary points that have yet, 40+ years later, to be fully addressed (indeed active disengagement has occurred). The problems with what is now termed 'lifestyle drift' in policy are introduced. These types of policies up front exhort concerns with taking on structural social issues to address equity, but then direct actions to individual behaviour and individual responsibility. Cautioning against the danger of 'excessive definitional breadth' is also raised when the core framing focus ought to be on 'crass-materialism' (p.258) that creates distributive health inequities. Addressing these inequities requires 'addressing the criteria and processes by which complex and difficult trade-offs should be made' (p. 259). This is followed by three truisms core for HPP: 'public health has always been political' (p. 259), 'A healthy lifestyle is an almost irrelevant concept in an unhealthy environment' (p. 260) and a quote from the political scientist Charles Lindblom that corporations 'command more resources than most government units…insist that governments meet their demands, even if those demands are counter to those of citizens…They are on all counts disproportionately powerful' (p. 260).

Despite this notable scholarship in the late 1980s, HPP is not, however, a modern phenomenon (see also de Leeuw, 2017; McManus, 2022). Historically, public health policy, through social welfare, was embedded in the sixteenth-century Poor Laws (Szreter et al. 2016). The mid-nineteenth-century environmental and urban health concerns that were at the core of public health legislation in England were an early example of HPP (Milio, 2001; Szreter, 2005). Both, the historian Simon Szreter has shown, came about in response to societal conditions related to urbanisation to address poverty and public health. Crucially, Szreter's analysis shows that these policy interventions are necessary for societies to function both socially *and* economically.

At the same time, in France, an explicit connection between health hazards and the 'mouvement hygieneste' underpinned the First Urban Planning Act Prohibiting the Rent of Substandard Housing (Jordan, 1995). That involved the commissioning of Pierre Haussmann to design Parisian infrastructure into the grand boulevards that city remains famous for today (de Leeuw, 2017).

Enter the original 'healthy urbanist', Edwin Chadwick. Chadwick was the architect of nineteenth-century public health legislation in England to address poverty through sanitation (Acheson, 1990). The period of activity preceding that legislation has been described as possibly the most successful instance of public health policy in the history of public health (Hamlin & Sidley, 1998). Essentially, Hamlin and Sidley show, the work was proactive rather than reactive, and politically and technically adept— Chadwick, the authors enthuse, 'transformed policy analysis'—by aiming squarely at the structures that create ill health in populations. Influence also occurred over a long period of time.

Around the same time the German physician Rudolf Virchow famously linked public health with social and economic conditions, subsequently serving as a politician to advance a essentially public health agenda (Schultz, 2008). Fast forward to 1920 and we find C-E A Winslow, a bacteriologist and public health expert, writing 'If it is good public policy to provide for the school child whatever machinery is necessary to make possible the attainment of a reasonable standard of physical health, it is difficult to see why the same argument does not apply to the adult as well' (p. 27) (Winslow, 1920). However, despite these achievements, it is important to recognise that linking health to societal conditions remained institutionally marginal rather than mainstream 'in the face of Cartesian, reductionist, and structural-biomedical approaches' (De Leeuw, 2017, p. 10).

'Healthy Public Policy' was given its modern impetus through the 'Ottawa Charter for Health Promotion' (World Health Organization, 1986). What is sometimes forgotten in the quest for HPP is how the Ottawa Charter itself focussed on different types of 'health promotion action'. The first two types are the most important for this book and are shown in Box 2.1 (the other levels being 'strengthen community actions', 'develop personal skills' and 'reorient health services').

Box 2.1: Ottawa charter Building HPP and Creating Supportive Environments
https://www.who.int/healthpromotion/conferences/previous/ottawa/en/index1.html Health Promotion Action Means:

Build Healthy Public Policy
Health promotion goes beyond health care. It puts health on the agenda of policy makers in all sectors and at all levels, directing them to be

aware of the health consequences of their decisions and to accept their responsibilities for health.

Health promotion policy combines diverse but complementary approaches including legislation, fiscal measures, taxation and organizational change. It is coordinated action that leads to health, income and social policies that foster greater equity. Joint action contributes to ensuring safer and healthier goods and services, healthier public services, and cleaner, more enjoyable environments.

Health promotion policy requires the identification of obstacles to the adoption of healthy public policies in non-health sectors, and ways of removing them. The aim must be to make the healthier choice the easier choice for policy makers as well.

Create Supportive Environments

Our societies are complex and interrelated. Health cannot be separated from other goals. The inextricable links between people and their environment constitutes the basis for a socioecological approach to health. The overall guiding principle for the world, nations, regions and communities alike, is the need to encourage reciprocal maintenance—to take care of each other, our communities and our natural environment. The conservation of natural resources throughout the world should be emphasized as a global responsibility.

Changing patterns of life, work and leisure have a significant impact on health. Work and leisure should be a source of health for people. The way society organizes work should help create a healthy society. Health promotion generates living and working conditions that are safe, stimulating, satisfying and enjoyable.

Systematic assessment of the health impact of a rapidly changing environment—particularly in areas of technology, work, energy production and urbanization—is essential and must be followed by action to ensure positive benefit to the health of the public. The protection of the natural and built environments and the conservation of natural resources must be addressed in any health promotion strategy.

Health in All Policies or Healthy Public Policy?

In recent years, there has been some confusion about whether Health in All Policies (HiAP) replaces HPP. There has been very good writing about HiAP that is highly relevant to HPP action. But HiAP, along with intersectoral action, is best understood as one recent strategy to achieve HPP (Friel et al., 2015; Lawless et al. 2017). In and of itself, HiAP has been shown to lack clarity of purpose and thus risk ineffectiveness as a body of policy action (Cairney et al., 2021).

The misnaming of HiAP is problematic because it presents the assumption that public policymakers—education, housing, urban and so forth—will have an innate interest in health. History shows that assumption to be incorrect. Today, given that 'health(care)' sucks up a large proportion of the public purse, it is even more problematic to emphasise. I prefer the longer used HPP. HPP at least connects, as introduced above, with the known dimensions of public policy that have been around since the middle of the last century.

For me, two critical differences between Healthy Public Policy (HPP) and Health in All Policies (HiAP) are that:

- HPP emphasises the many and varied connections between public policy and health, and aims to influence public policy to be 'healthy' from an institutional perspective and not necessarily driven by health advocates; and
- HiAP is a sub-strategy of HPP, most often led by health advocates but emphasising collaboration with other sectors, that aims to work across sectors from whatever leverage point that makes it possible to include 'health' in any policy at any level for any organisation or community.

Urban Healthy Public Policy

This history outlined in this chapter has already hinted at how HPP has often come about with an urban lens. A good example is the 'healthy cities' movement and its many cross-overs with HPP. Healthy cities arose around the same time as the Ottawa Charter and have inextricable conceptual links that connect HPP with the creation of supportive environments. De Leeuw, introducing healthy cities, provides an informative historical timeline to the relationship between cities and human health (de Leeuw, 2017). Historical human settlement patterns, she explains, and increasing urbanisation, led to the various 'epidemiological transitions' that characterise human progress. Our history includes not only the causes of human health but the responses to protect and promote health—not necessarily public policy responses but certainly early pre-cursors. For instance, water management systems were established 4000 years ago in Mesopotamia. 'The connection' De Leeuw writes, 'between health and urban planning has therefore always existed, implicitly or explicitly' (p. 9). Importantly, healthy cities practitioners have a complex view of the relationship between health and the urban form: cities are 'best understood holistically, as an organic, living system, partly organism, partly ecosystem' (p. 9). The core dynamics of a 'healthy city' are listed in Box 2.2. Many of these, I contend, lay the foundations for the importance of public policy that is 'healthy'.

Box 2.2: Core dynamics behind Healthy Cities (De Leeuw, 2012)
Two of the original architects of the 'healthy cities' movement, Trevor Hancock and Leonard Duhl, proposed, at the launch of the "official" WHO Healthy Cities Project in 1986, the following 11 parameters for a Healthy City:

1. A clean, safe, high-quality physical environment (including housing quality)
2. An ecosystem which is stable now and sustainable in the long-term
3. A strong, mutually supportive and non-exploitive community
4. A high degree of public participation in and control over the decisions affecting one's life, health, and well-being
5. The meeting of basic needs (food, water, shelter, income, safety, and work) for all the city's people
6. Access to a wide variety of experiences and resources with the possibility of multiple contacts, interaction, and communication
7. A diverse, vital, and innovative city economy
8. Encouragement of connectedness with the past, with the cultural and biological heritage, and with other groups and individuals
9. A city form that is compatible with and enhances the above parameters and behaviours
10. An optimum level of appropriate public-health and sick-care services accessible to all
11. High health status (both high positive health status and low disease status)

Healthy cities is also innovative for its embrace of politics. In an excellent historical introduction to 'City Planning', Corburn (2017a, 2017b) explains how the initial nineteenth-century connections between health and planning systems were lost as scientific methodological reductionism took hold in the twentieth century. Reductionist thinking, Corburn argues, is the reason that 'health' became medicalised, and cities became managed and planned through separate professionally differentiated municipal bureaucracies including water, housing, transport and so forth. In a similar argument to the technical vs strategic nature of public health policy, introduced earlier in this chapter, Corburn finds much writing on urban health to be apolitical. He explains, for example, how the typical framing of 'the built environment and health' tends to ignore the politics of urban and regional planning. This avoidance of politics, he argues, is to the detriment of both sectors effectively addressing 'the root causes of poor health, not just to devise interventions aimed at specific diseases or individual behaviours'.

My work is, I hope, an extension of this type of 'healthy city' thinking.

Equity as the Goal for Healthy Public Policy: 'Place' as a Working Example

For public health advocates of HPP progressing action to improve health equity is an essential value and interest. Indeed, much of the effort behind HPP is about equity. That goal is important to understand, especially for those readers who may not be familiar with why public health people are interested in other people's disciplines or areas of policymaking. Here, I take an urban flavour to health equity, zeroing in on a strand of literature that focusses on the relationship of 'places' to health equity. This is largely because I return to that problem of 'place-making' in the latter parts of the book.

Urban 'places' in cities and regions influence health equity through the decisions that are made about the provision of built and social infrastructure (Macintyre et al., 2002). 'Place-based' interventions are known to be effective in improving health (Arcaya et al. 2016; McGowan et al. 2021). The influence of place on health is *relational*, resulting from the interaction of people with the wider environment (Cummins et al. 2007). One of my favourite titles of a recent book is Clare Bambra's 'Health Divides: where you live can kill you' (Bambra, 2016). Bambra demonstrates how differences in places and spaces—where people live—result in unfair and inequitable differences in health status. Focussing on cities for example, health is inequitably distributed by socio-economic status and area level disadvantage (Litman, 2013; Giles-Corti et al. 2016). In countries like Australia, for instance, suburbia tends to be more disadvantaged with worse health status compared to inner regions and urban centres, largely explained by infrastructural investments favouring the latter (Arundel et al., 2017).

Health (in)equity is defined as the unfair and avoidable difference in health between groups and populations (Dahlgren, 1991). Importantly, both conceptually and for action, addressing health equity requires a *relational* approach to considering urban places (Corburn, 2017a, 2017b; Healey, 2006). Given that fairness an essential ingredient HPP for equity also means focussing on actions to address or redress those inequities. That relational approach is not only about the known links between inequity created by a mix of composition—the people who live there—or contextual—the environment surrounding people (Cummins et al., 2007). Concentrations of disadvantage in certain places are the result of a complex mix of social, spatial, economic and political forces (Bambra, 2016; Larsen, 2007; Rushton, 2014). The emphasis must be on interplays, *across and within* an urban area, of economic, socio-cultural, environmental *and*, for the purposes of this book, political/administrative dynamics (Corburn, 2009, 2017a, 2017b). As I go on to show at length, understanding and acting on relational place-making for (health and social) equity emphasises the wielding of power by way of policy, by policymakers, and whether power is shared or held (Corburn, 2017a, 2017b; Friel et al. 2021; Fincher et al., 2016; Harris et al. 2020).

Conclusion: Evidence 'of Policy'

This chapter has introduced the history of HPP and provided insights to what HPP looks like, especially from an 'urban' historical perspective. In doing so, the chapter has articulated the intent of HPP and, by extension, this book, to understand the dynamics of public health policy. This task is, I have shown, both technical and strategic. Public health is political. It is only by embracing the core of what 'Public policy' is that progress towards a healthier and more equitable society can be made.

I want to close this chapter with a brief observation about evidence. Apart from my introduction, above, to the evidence about health equity and place, evidence has thus far only been an undercurrent to the narrative. Just as the literature I have introduced here is vast, so is the evidence base about the health effects of policy. Indeed, much of that literature today tends to present that vast evidence base as ideas 'for' policymakers to take on. The greatest success of the World Health Organisation's Commission on the Social Determinants of Health, for example, was to provide a comprehensive evidence base about health inequity (World Health Organisation, 2008). The result of the Commission's intentional avoidance of politics led to accusations of insufficient articulation of what was needed for change to occur (Navarro, 2009). Similarly, but more recently, comprehensive evidence linking cities with human health was reviewed for a 2016 Lancet Commission (Giles-Corti et al., 2016). As an example of why technical presentation of evidence is important but insufficient for action, this body of work recommends 'integrated planning' of cities to link up siloed decision-making. Despite that exhortation, the papers avoid mention of the politics that sit behind making integrated planning work or not. I address these politics head on in the second part of this book.

That said, there will always be a need to provide robust evidence of the problems that need HPP action. My respect for those who have demonstrated evidence of impact knows no bounds. There is a truism to the notion that policymakers want researchers to show them the numbers. However, the premise of this book is that there is insufficient attention on policymaking as the point at which the evidence either is or is not taken up. The challenge, in my view, laid down by both HPP and related movements like healthy cities is to accept the evidence and take action to change policy (Atkinson, 2015; Bambra et al., 2005; Raphael, 2014; Milio, 1987). Put simply, evidence alone is insufficient for policy influence (Fafard, 2015, Fafard et al., 2021).

Fortunately, work in political science and allied disciplines already provides a comprehensive and sophisticated understanding of the role that scientific evidence does and does not play in policymaking. This extends to include research on policymaking in cities. Both bodies of work consistently demonstrate how evidence generation is but one consideration among many in policy and politics. Turning this argument back in on itself, translating evidence 'for policy' into policymaking requires a sound understanding 'of policy' processes and institutions. The next chapter explains how to go about generating the evidence 'about policy'.

REFERENCES

Acheson, D. (1990). Edwin Chadwick and the world we live in. *The Lancet*, *336*(8729), 1482–1485.

Arcaya, M. C., et al. (2016). Research on neighborhood effects on health in the United States: A systematic review of study characteristics. *Social Science & Medicine, 168*, 16–29.

Arts, B., & Van Tatenhove, J. (2004). Policy and power: A conceptual framework between the 'old'and 'new'policy idioms. *Policy Sciences, 37*(3–4), 339–356.

Arundel, J., Lowe M., & H. P. (2017). *Creating liveable cities in Australia Mapping urban policy implementation and evidence-based national liveability indicators*. RMIT Centre for Urban Research.

Atkinson, A. B. (2015). *Inequality*. Harvard University Press.

Bambra, C. (2016). *Health divides: Where you live can kill you*. Policy Press.

Bambra, C., Fox, D., & Scott-Samuel, A. (2005). Towards a politics of health. *Health Promotion International, 20*(2), 187–193.

Bambra, C., Lynch J., & Smith, K. E. (2021). *The unequal pandemic: COVID-19 and health inequalities*. Policy Press.

Cairney, P., St Denny, E., & Mitchell, H. (2021). *The future of public health policymaking after COVID-19: A qualitative systematic review of lessons from Health in All Policies. Open Research Europe, 1*, 23.

Carstensen, M. B., & Schmidt, V. A. (2016). Power through, over and in ideas: Conceptualizing ideational power in discursive institutionalism. *Journal of European Public Policy, 23*(3), 318–337.

Corburn, J. (2017a). Equitable and healthy city planning: Towards healthy urban governance in the century of the city. *Healthy Cities* (pp. 31–41). Springer.

Corburn, J. (2009). *Toward the healthy city: People, places, and the politics of urban planning*. MIT Press.

Corburn, J. (2017b). Urban place and health equity: Critical issues and practices. *International Journal of Environmental Research and Public Health, 14*(2), 117.

Cummins, S., Curtis, S., Diez-Roux, A. V., & Macintyre, S. (2007). *Understanding and representing 'place' in health research: A relational approach. Social Science & Medicine, 65*(9), 1825–1838.

Dahlgren, G., & Whitehead, M. (1991). *Policies and strategies to promote social equity in health*. Institute for Future Studies.

de Leeuw, E. (2017). Cities and health from the neolithic to the Anthropocene. *Healthy Cities* (pp. 3–30). Springer.

De Leeuw, E. (2012). Do healthy cities work? A logic of method for assessing impact and outcome of healthy cities. *Journal of Urban Health, 89*(2), 217–231.

De Leeuw, E., & Harris, P. (2022). Governance and policies for setings based work. In S. Kokko (Ed.), *Handbook of settings based health promotion*. Springer Nature.

Fafard, P. (2015). Beyond the usual suspects: Using political science to enhance public health policy making. *JECH, 69*(11), 1129–1132.

Fincher, R., Pardy, M., & Shaw, K. (2016). Place-making or place-masking? The everyday political economy of "making place." *Planning Theory and Practice, 17*(4), 516–536.

Friel, S., Harris, P., Simpson, S., Bhushan, A., Baer, B. (2015). *Health in all policies approaches: Pearls from the Western Pacific Region. Asia & the Pacific Policy Studies, 2*(2): 324–337.

Friel, S., Townsend, B., Fisher, M., Harris, P., Freeman, T., & Baum, F. J. (2021, August). Power and the people's health. *Social Science and Medicine, 282,* 114173.

Giles-Corti, B., et al. (2016). City planning and population health: A global challenge. *The Lancet, 388*(10062), 2912–2924.

Hamlin, C., & Sidley, P. (1998). Revolutions in public health: 1848, and 1998? *BMJ, 317*(7158), 587.

Hancock, T. (1985). Beyond health care: From public health policy to healthy public policy. *Canadian Journal of Public Health, 76*(Suppl 1), 9–11.

Harris, P., Baum, F., Friel, S., Mackean, T., Schram, A., & Townsend, B. (2020). A glossary of theories for understanding power and policy for health equity. *Journal of Epidemiology and Community Health, 74,* 548–552.

Harris, P. J., Kemp, L. A., & Sainsbury, P. (2012). The essential elements of health impact assessment and healthy public policy: A qualitative study of practitioner perspectives. *British Medical Journal Open, 2*(6), e001245.

Healey, P. (2006). *Urban complexity and spatial strategies: Towards a relational planning for our times.* Routledge.

Howarth, D. (2010). Power, discourse, and policy: Articulating a hegemony approach to critical policy studies. *Critical Policy Studies, 3*(3–4), 309–335.

Howlett, M., Ramesh, M., & Perl, A. (2009). *Studying public policy: Policy cycles and policy sub-systems* (3rd ed.). Oxford University Press.

Jordan, D. P. (1995). *Transforming Paris: The life and labors of Baron Haussman.* Simon and Schuster.

Larsen, K. (2007). *The health impacts of place-based interventions in areas of concentrated disadvantaged: A review of literature.* Sydney South West Area Health Service, NSW Health.

Laumann, E. O., & Knoke, D. (1987). *The organizational state: Social choice in national policy domains.* University of Wisconsin Press.

Lawless, A. P., Baum, F., Delany-Crowe, T., MacDougall, C., Williams, C., McDermott, D., & van Eyk, H. (2017). Developing a framework for a program theory-based approach to evaluating policy processes and outcomes: Health in all policies in South Australia. *International Journal of Health Policy and Management, 7*(6), 510–521.

Litman, T. (2013). Transportation and public health. *Annual Review of Public Health, 34,* 217–233.

Macintyre, S., Ellaway, A., & Cummins, S. (2002). Place effects on health: How can we conceptualise, operationalise and measure them? *Social Science & Medicine, 55*(1), 125–139.

McGowan, V.J., Buckner, S., Mead, R., McGill, E., Ronzi, S., Beyer, F., & Bambra, C. (2021). Examining the effectiveness of place-based interventions to improve public health and reduce health inequalities: An umbrella review. *BMC Public Health, 21*(1), 1–17.

McManus, P. (2022). Infrastructure, health and urban planning: Rethinking the past and exploring future possibilities. *Infrastructure and Health* (In press).

Milio, N. (2001). Glossary: Healthy public policy. *Journal of Epidemiology & Community Health, 55*(9), 622–623.

Milio, N. (1987). Making healthy public policy; developing the science by learning the art: An ecological framework for policy studies. *Health Promotion International, 2*(3), 263–274.

Milio, N. (1981). *Promoting health through public policy.* Davis.

Navarro, V. (2009). What we mean by social determinants of health. *J International Journal of Health Services, 39*(3), 423–441.

Raphael, D. (2014). Beyond policy analysis: The raw politics behind opposition to healthy public policy. *Health Promotion International, 30*(2), 380–396.

Rein, M., & Schön, D. (1994). *Frame reflection: Toward the resolution of intractable policy controversies.* Basic Book.

Rushton, C. (2014). Whose place is it anyway? Representational politics in a place-based health initiative. *Health & Place, 26*, 100–109.

Sabatier, P. A. (1988). An advocacy coalition framework of policy change and the role of policy-oriented learning therein. *Policy Sciences, 21*(2), 129–168.

Schmidt, V. A. (2008). Discursive institutionalism: The explanatory power of ideas and discourse. *Annual Review of Political Science, 11*, 303–326.

Schultz, M. (2008). Rudolf Virchow. *Emerging Infectious Diseases, 14*(9), 1480.

Smith, K. (2013). *Beyond evidence based policy in public health: The interplay of ideas.* Springer.

Stone, D.A. (1997). *Policy paradox: The art of political decision making* (Vol. 13). W. W .Norton.

Szreter, S., et al. (2016). Health, welfare, and the state—the dangers of forgetting history. *The Lancet, 388*(10061), 2734–2735.

Szreter, S. (2005). *Health and wealth studies in history and policy* (Vol. 6). Boydell and Brewer.

Tesh, S., Tuohy, C., Christoffel, T., Hancock, T., Norsigian, J., Nightingale, E., & Robertson, L. (1987). The meaning of healthy public policy. *Health Promotion International, 2*(3), 257–262.

Williams, S. J. (2003). Beyond meaning, discourse and the empirical world: Critical realist reflections on health. *Social Theory & Health, 1*, 42–71.

Winslow, C.-E. (1920). *The untilled fields of public health. Science, 51*, 23–33.

World Health Organisation. (2008). *Closing the gap in a generation: Health equity through action on the social determinants of health* (Final Report of the Commission on Social Determinants of Health). World Health Organization.

World Health Organization. (1986). *Ottawa charter for health promotion.*

CHAPTER 3

Healthy Public Policy Analysis: Switching on the Floodlights

Before starting any research enterprise, it is crucial to ask what type of knowledge we want to produce. This chapter introduces philosophical and methodological underpinnings of a critical social science approach to researching public health policy. The focal point is the everyday, often complex, world of policymaking. Critical realism is the body of knowledge I draw on here as my methodological underpinning.

Forewarned is forearmed. We're exploring at the deepest, abstracted, point of the book here. The language is slippery, and the ideas presented at their densest. But like most endeavours, navigating these depths are necessary to glean a proper understanding. Note my attempt throughout to keep it light while retaining depth. Not an easy task. I'll start that attempt with an analogy about floodlights.

The best description of the intent of this type of research comes from a colleague of mine working in infrastructure in Australia (Gary Bowditch). Professor Bowditch once wryly observed to me that what is required to understand infrastructure policy and practice is research that 'uses floodlights instead of microscopes'. This sentiment is no stranger to urban researchers. For instance, the pioneering urban geographer David Harvey (Harvey, 1987)—whose work this book returns to often—similarly explains his approach:

P. Harris, *Illuminating Policy for Health*, Palgrave Studies in Public Health Policy Research, https://doi.org/10.1007/978-3-031-13199-8_3

Marx's[1] objective in Capital (page 19) is to "lay bare the economic law of motion" of capitalism. Since neither "microscopes nor chemical reagents are of use," the "force of abstraction must replace both. (p. 372)

As Harvey suggests, choosing floodlights over microscopes is a philosophical question. Answering that question requires differentiating between ontology (what reality is) and epistemology (how we can know reality) as well as methodology (how we go about studying reality). Abstraction, just as Harvey exhorts, is the task that allows a researcher to straddle across and jump between these different analytic points.

CRITICAL REALISM

Critical realism (CR) builds from the acceptance that the choice of research design hinges on questions about the nature of reality—ontology—and how we gain knowledge about reality—epistemology—(Danermark et al., 2002; Mingers, 2014). Ontology is a word that strikes confusion in the heart of many a researcher, impenetrable at best, irrelevant at worst. 'Not so!', CR philosophers exclaim, who argue that ontology is the route to understanding the complex nature of reality itself (Collier, 1994; Outhwaite, 1987; Potter & Lopez, 2001; Sayer, 2000).

CRists[2] tend to pitch themselves against two principle 'meta-theories' of social science: positivism and relativism (Danermark et al., 2002). A lot of this CR writing sets up 'straw man' arguments to explain the core differences between CR and other more standard[3] knowledge paradigms. An unfortunate consequence, however, is the suggestion that CR offers insights that other approaches to research cannot. Such dogmatic ownership of methodology is a weakness because it sets CR up as an outsider to knowledge and practice (Mingers, 2014).

---

[1] In case any readers, especially from Public Health, balk at the Marxian method, please refer to the excellent introductory exhortation to really understand and use Marx's method by none other than the Editor in Chief of The Lancet: Horton, R. (2017). Offline: Medicine and Marx. *Lancet, 390,* 20,126.

[2] In my opinion, one of the clearest writers about critical realism is Andrew Sayer. Sayer, an urban geographer by core discipline, will be familiar to urbanist readers (the connections between urbanism and critical realism are long and deep).

[3] Roy Bhaskar, one of the main architects of the critical realist approach, was not part of the formal university 'Academy' system (see Mingers, 2014).

According to CR, both positivism and postmodernism share over-reliance on empiricism in social science. This is coined 'the epistemic fallacy': positivism and relativism mix up and thereby join together (otherwise called 'conflating') the relationship between the nature of objects, ontology, with the social knowledge of them, epistemology (Bhaskar, 1978). The result of the epistemic fallacy is that, rather than seeking depth, the practice of science is conflated with the underlying reality of being, 'as if the world just happened to correspond to the range of our senses and to be identical to what we experience' (Sayer, 2000, p. 11).

The epistemic fallacy is no stranger to health (promotion) researchers who will be familiar with the institutionalised adage that methods drive research rather than the other way round. McQueen and Anderson, in their classic text about health promotion[4] evaluation, take a similar line. They complain about researchers putting 'methodology' over and above the use of theory and models for advancing knowledge (McQueen & Anderson, 2001, p. 73). Similarly, De Leeuw in her healthy cities work describes how the wrong choice of research design, driven by concerns over methods and whether journals will publish the paper or not, results in various 'error types' (De Leeuw, 2012). Error type III occurs, she contends, when the research design answers the wrong question: ('Why are there more hospital beds in Healthy Cities' for instance). Error type IV is more pernicious, she argues, in that it corresponds to answering the right question from the wrong paradigm: ('An investigation of Healthy City governance using an experimental research design' is De Leeuw's example).

Avoiding such errors requires maintaining 'the independence of the world from our thoughts about it' (Sayer, 2000, p. 10). A helpful CR strategy is to differentiate between the object of science and the practice of science (Collier, 1994; Danermark et al., 2002; Sayer, 2000). Like the core tenet of positivism, the goal is to capture what is real but stands apart from our subjective understanding of what we are researching. The separation of fact from reality will, however, rile up relativists, whom CRists call 'hard constructivists', because relativists tend to suggest that separating ontology (reality) from research is not possible and therefore of no interest—see for instance (Baert, 2005).

---

[4] For non-Public Health folk, Health Promotion is a sub-discipline of Public Health. Note that the Ottawa Charter, introduced last chapter, is foundational for Health Promotion.

Most CR research, including that presented in this book, conforms to 'soft constructivism' (Marsh, 2009; Sayer, 2000). Soft constructivism takes the position that social reality is constructed, but it also has real effects. Knowledge of something can never really be objectively separated from that something. Even the best designed randomised control trial is based on a set of assumptions about reality, for instance. Away from research designs, policymaking practice and policy systems are easier examples of social constructivism. Policy is largely socially constructed (Marsh, 2009). Policymaking can never being truly separate from our knowledge of it (indeed politics thrives on the connections to subjective knowledge).

The final point all this philosophising comes to is the notion of what is real or what is 'the truth'. To do this, CR emphasises both *fallibility* and *practical adequacy*. For CR, explanations from research are fallible and, over time, may require change or refinement if they are to adequately explain the object of interest (Sayer, 2000). Descriptions, or discourses, are culturally and historically situated and are fallible because they are human (Potter & Lopez, 2001). Nevertheless, for CRists, some explanations are better than others and can be judged as such. Given that absolute truth is ultimately unobtainable (Outhwaite, 1987; Pratt, 1995), the goal of science for CRists is the 'practical adequacy' of explanations in terms of their connection with the real world.

A similar concept, proposed by DeLeeuw in the healthy cities literature (De Leeuw, 2009; de Leeuw & Skovgaard, 2005), is 'utility-driven evidence'. The essential question is how does knowledge produced by research shape good practice and guide policy decisions (De Leeuw, 2009, p. i21)?

To that end, CR is no different from other science. The task of science is to apply a rigorous systematic approach that is communicated via a decent readable narrative (Savage & Yeh, 2019). Much CR writing, however, fails on the narrative front.

What Does Reality Look like?

At the epicentre of CR research is the search for underlying mechanisms that make things happen in reality. The whole purpose of science is to *'investigate and identify relationships and non-relationships respectively, between what we experience, what actually happens, and the underlying*

Table 3.1 Domains of Reality (Adapted from Bhaskar, 1978; Collier, 1994)

	Domain of the real	Domain of the actual	Domain of the empirical
Mechanism/structure	✓		
Events	✓	✓	
Experiences	✓	✓	✓

mechanisms that produce the events in the world' (Danermark et al., 2002, p. 21: italics in original).

One does not just stumble upon these deeper explanations of reality. Rather, as the above quote suggests, there are layers of analysis which establish depth to reality (Collier, 1994, p. 42). CR's principal architect, Roy Bhaskar, came up with the three domains that the realist enterprise aims to uncover. These domains are shown in Table 3.1, named by Bhaskar (1978) as 'the real', 'the actual' and 'the empirical'.

A brief introduction to each domain is required. The 'real' domain refers to deep underlying mechanisms and entities, and the structure and the power of objects (Outhwaite, 1987; Sayer, 2000; Williams, 2003). The real contains generative causal mechanisms which exist *independent of* our knowledge or sense perception of them (Williams, 2003). Thus, identifying these mechanisms 'means shifting attention to what produces events – not just the events themselves' (Danermark et al., 2002, p. 5). These events, and our experiences of them, are what 'the actual' domain is made up of (Collier, 1994; Outhwaite, 1987; Williams, 2003). The 'actual' concerns the activation of the structures and powers of the real, what happens if and when these are activated, what they do and what eventuates when they do (Sayer, 2000). The third domain, the empirical domain, is made up of observable experiences (Collier, 1994; Outhwaite, 1987; Williams, 2003).

My view is that the column on the left of Table 3.1 is iterative and joined to the others. As I go on to show, explanations of structures and mechanisms can, indeed should, be rooted in the language of and insights from practical, lived, experience. I will repeat myself ad nauseum about this throughout the book: both empirical data and theoretical explanation join to create knowledge about reality.

Just in case this has been missed, empirical data are emphasised as essential in critical realist research (Sayer, 1998) and fundamental to the policy analysis approach presented in this book. The grounding of the research in empirical evidence, according to Danermark et al. (2002), is important, 'so that abstractions do not occur in a vacuum' (p. 62). Similarly, Sayer cautions that over-reliance on theoretical abstraction without empirical observation of the concrete leads to 'pseudo-concrete' research that over-emphasises 'big theories' at the expense of reality (Sayer, 1992). Similarly, Layder argues for 'empirically anchoring' (1998, p. 113) research where the data provide the categorical, 'practically adequate' entry point into the phenomena.

To sum up, the mixing of empirical and theoretical analysis is fundamental to turning on the floodlights in policy research. At the centre of this type of analysis is the task of abstraction.

The Task of Abstraction

CR analysis has at its core a movement from empirical data about experience to theoretical abstraction and back again. This iterative—back and forth—movement is 'Abstraction' (Collier, 1994; Danermark et al., 2002; Layder, 1998; Ollman, 2001; Outhwaite, 1987; Sayer, 1992, 1998, 2000; Stones, 1996). Returning to the three stratified levels of reality, the main purpose of abstraction is to isolate causal and generative mechanisms and structures which occur at the level of 'the real' (Yeung, 1997).

Abstraction in CR is very similar to what other scientific approaches call 'inferential processes' (Downward et al., 2002; Potter & Lopez, 2001). Inference, the process of formulating and assessing the reliability of knowledge claims—rather than logical deduction or numerical probabilities—provides the rigour in CR research (Downward et al., 2002). Crucially, observation and theory are equal (Danermark et al., 2002).

Abstraction is at the heart of two formal steps unique to the CR endeavour, 'abduction' and 'retroduction'—themselves a step in the analysis I present next chapter. The central task is to shift knowledge of some phenomenon of interest to the mechanisms, structures or conditions responsible for that phenomenon. In essence, the move is from a surface view of something to a deeper explanation of that same thing (Lawson, 2003), p. 145).

The concept of 'shuttling between' (Layder, 1998, p. 108) abstract and concrete reasoning explains the task of abstraction. An abstraction is something that is formed when we separate or isolate in thought one particular aspect of a concrete phenomenon or object (Danermark et al., 2002; Sayer, 1992). Concrete, as the name suggests, covers empirical data about the social world and our experience of it. Abstracting moves away from that data to a higher order, usually theory (Sayer, 1992, p. 116). Essentially, the task is to see what the core dimensions of some phenomenon is, break the phenomenon apart, peer underneath to see what the causes are and then come up with a complete explanation.

The ability to shuttle between the abstract and the concrete requires creativity. Intuition, perception and sensitivity or readiness represent a 'predisposition to 'lock-on' to suggestive ideas and concepts (Layder, 1998, p. 107). The process is initially chaotic, but by taking a systematic approach it is possible to combine abstractions to form concepts which 'grasp the concreteness of their objects' (Sayer, 1992, p. 87).

Similar points about science and abstraction have been made in the political science and urban studies literature. In political science, Paul Cairney has called for reinvigorated focus on using the intersections between multiple theories to explain real-world instances of policymaking (Cairney, 2013; Weible, 2014). Cairney (2013) makes some excellent observations about different methodologies and ontologies. He argues that a 'complementary' approach where theory is used iteratively to explain data is often more useful for policy analysis than traditional positivist or empiricist-driven approaches.

Urban studies is also no stranger to abstraction. The Harvey (1987) quote at the start of this chapter comes from a foundational debate in the journal 'Environment and Planning D: Society and Space' about the position of social theory in urban and regional research and analysis. Harvey does two important things with his argument. First, he explains the importance of abstraction as an urban research method. Second, he questions whether the realist method tips the balance towards data rather than theory. His point is that over-reliance on empirical data avoids critical analysis and indeed may perpetuate the problems in society that research is meant to critique and change—capitalism looms large of course. In the debate that follows, several urban thinkers and researchers then run with this argument. Some support but ask important questions about the realist agenda. Then, our old CR friend Andrew Sayer has his say.

For me, the debate turns on what realist abstraction is in practice. Sayer's main point in his conclusion (and later work) seals, for me, the debate. Abstraction, as realists practice it, moves between data and theory in a manner that is not only deductive (theory driven) or inductive (data driven). It is not one or the other but a mix of both.

This debate about theorising has special relevance to policy analysis. Does all analysis of policy really need to be about political economy? What if the focus is not on urban life in its totality but on the process of urban and regional policymaking? There are a great many theories about policy that are required to understand how policy is made and under what conditions. Harvey's use of Marx is great for the macro but not so useful for the micro, for instance. This point is taken up strongly in the debate by the (since very successful urban scholar) Michael Storper (1987) in his response to Harvey:

> The most fertile work in Marxist political economy recently has used a sensitive and flexible application of mesolevel theoretical constructs which focus on social organization in relation to politics and economics. (p. 423)

Since that time, critical (realist) urbanists like Neil Brenner are clearer about analysing being a mix of abstraction—theory—and concrete—data (Brenner, 2009, 2019). For example, Brenner (2019) provides a very useful roadmap under the pompously titled 'some distinctions for deciphering the contemporary mutations of the urban question' (p. 345). Like the realist analysis I describe here, Brenner articulates 'refining' concepts 'reflexively' via theory and data, and employing 'theoretical abstractions' to specify the 'essential properties of the urban (as an historically and geographically embedded') analytical object/site of investigation' (p. 345). Brenner then advocates for the ultimate extension of abstraction as 'transcending narrow city centric' epistemologies to embed the analysis in the multi-scalar political economy of the Capitalist urban fabric.

'Be still my beating heart!' I hear you mutter. Fear not. While I agree with about this laudable goal, not all of us are in the position to reach such starry heights. Research often depends not only on the question being asked but the capacity, resources and time available to get there. But what Brenner is essentially suggesting is to keep our abstracting eye on the 'multi-scalar' phenomenon of urban society. This, as I go on to show, is possible in most if not all research projects even without the funding for complex multi-country research projects.

Ok, time to stop and come up for air. At this point, you may well ask, 'but what has all this got to do with switching the floodlights on?'.

In sum, CR enables the search for floodlights precisely because CR analysis requires attending to conditions. Understanding and explaining those conditions, by switching on the floodlights, require abstracting out from empirical observation to a deeper theory of the wide range of mechanisms and structures. Two additional analytic tasks allow this to happen, looking for structures and working out causality.

Switching on the Floodlights

Here, I introduce the central analytic piece of the puzzle for policy research. Sayer (1992, 2000) proposes a series of questions for researchers to ask about the object of their investigation 'to sharpen our conceptualisations' (2000, p. 20), discover the structure of a system of interest (1992, p. 91) and thereby lessen the chance of misattribution. These questions form the basis of the 'retroduction' analytic stage introduced in the next chapter:

1. What does the existence of this object/practice presuppose? What are its preconditions?
2. Can/could object A exist without B? If not, what else must be present?
3. What is it about this object which enables it to do certain things (may be several mechanisms at work and need to seek ways to distinguish their respective efforts)?

Danermark et al. (2002) add a fourth question:

4. What cannot be removed without making the object cease to exist in its present form?

I came across these questions early in my policy research journey (Harris et al., 2012). I was at the time investigating how health impact assessment as a process intersects with policymaking. Using these questions, I was able to show how participants I had interviewed all pointed to public policy being core 'object' that needed better theorising to be understood. I then undertook that analysis with a new institutionalist lens (Harris, Sainsbury et al., 2014a, 2014b).

At a more substantive level, these questions are about relations between objects (Jessop, 1998). They are essentially qualitative rather than quantitative, in that they enable reasoning about the relational characteristics of objects rather than the regularities (Sayer, 2000). The next task, once the essentials are established, is to differentiate the relational dimensions between and among objects.

Enter the notions of 'contingency' and 'necessity'. A contingent relation in CR means that phenomena/objects of research under scrutiny might be related but do not necessarily depend on each other for their existence. Importantly, although a relation may be contingent, *it may still have significant effects* (Sayer, 2000, p. 89): hence the importance of planning for contingencies that might occur, but also might not, in major life decisions like building a house. In contrast, necessary relations between objects occur when the existence of one necessarily pre-supposes the other: the object is dependent on its relation to the other object.

When considering relations between objects, the essential emphasis is on causation, asking 'what causes one thing to lead to do something'. CR offers a framework for causal analysis in *social systems* (Mingers, 2014). Social systems are open rather than closed systems, and because of this concern relations over regularities. Regularities are the topic of Humean accounts of causation, which looks for 'constant conjunction' of observable events: whenever A occurs then B occurs. CR, instead, asks 'what is? That is, why does X behave the way it does, viz B, in conditions C1....Cn?' (Bhaskar, 1978, p. 172). Enter the term 'mechanism' which focusses attention on how objects work (Danermark et al., 2002).

As shown in Fig. 3.1, on the left to right diagonal, the structure of an object contains mechanisms which produce events. On the right to left diagonal, other objects contain mechanisms which become conditions influencing the mechanisms of the first object. Therein lies the switch to turn on the floodlights!

'Structure', as shown in Fig. 3.1, is at the heart of the object. Objects have the powers they have by virtue of their structures, and mechanisms exist and are what they are because of their structure: that is the nature of the object (Danermark et al., 2002). However, because open systems have structures that constantly interact, a multiplicity of mechanisms is in operation at different stratified levels (Sayer, 2000).

Powers and their tendencies lie beneath mechanisms. Mechanisms generally refer to how objects work. Mechanisms are dependent on the presence of conditions or circumstances that determine whether or not

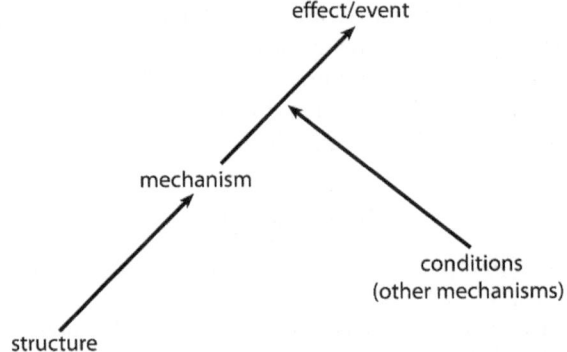

Fig. 3.1 Critical realist view of causation (Adapted from Sayer, 2000)

they will operate. Moreover, the events that are produced are also dependent on conditions. In other words, whether a causal power is actually activated or triggered depends on conditions (other mechanisms) whose presence and configuration are contingent, or external to the object (Danermark et al., 2002; Sayer, 1992). In this way, conditions are contextual manifestations that trigger whether mechanisms will result in an event or outcome (Pawson & Tilley, 1997). Conditions, along with structures, can be seen as triggers for mechanisms to become observable events.

SUMMARY

To summarise, this section has differentiated between CR as a meta-theory and analytic process. I have explained why critical realism as a meta-theory differs from both positivism and relativism, and in doing so set up its core elements. These are built on ontology (what we are able to know) being separated from epistemology (how we can know what we know). The search for this explanation looks for what is real at a level deeper than empiricism alone can allow for. As an analytic method, the task is to abstract between empiricism and theoretical explanation to arrive at more concrete explanations. Abstraction involves both structural and causal analysis where, because of the nature of open systems at the social level, causation searches for relations and not regularities.

That, then, is the way that CR enables researchers or analysts to switch on the floodlights. However, while the analytic process is set up, it is made easier by some type of isolation of the essential factors of the phenomenon under investigation. Fortunately for health focussed policy analysis, these essential characteristics are already provided. There are regular units of analysis that make up policy and policymaking. These units of analysis are the focus of Chapter 5. Before then, in the next chapter, I detail critical realist analysis as a set of systematic steps.

REFERENCES

Archer, M. S. (1995). *Realist social theory: The morphogenetic approach*. Cambridge University Press.

Arts, B., & Van Tatenhove, J. (2004). Policy and power: A conceptual framework between the 'old'and 'new'policy idioms. *Policy Sciences, 37*(3–4), 339–356.

Baert, P. (2005). *Philosophy of the social sciences: Towards pragmatism*. Polity.

Bhaskar, R. (1978). *A realist theory of science* (3rd ed.). New York, Verso.

Bilodeau, A., & Potvin, L. (2018). Unpacking complexity in public health interventions with the Actor-Network Theory. *Health Promotion International, 33*(1), 173–181.

Brenner, N. (2009). What is critical urban theory? *City, 13*(2–3), 198–207.

Brenner, N. (2019). *New urban spaces: Urban theory and the scale question*. Oxford University Press.

Cairney, P. (2011). *Understanding public policy: Theories and issues*. Palgrave Macmillan.

Cairney, P. (2013). Standing on the shoulders of giants: How do we combine the insights of multiple theories in public policy studies? *Policy Studies Journal, 41*(1), 1–21.

Cairney, P., St Denny, E., & Mitchell, H. (2021). The future of public health policymaking after COVID-19: A qualitative systematic review of lessons from Health in All Policies. *Open Research Europe, 1*, 23.

Clarke, S. E. (2015). Emerging research agendas. In K. Mossberger, S. E. Clarke, & P. John (Eds.), *The Oxford handbook of urban politics*.

Clegg, S. R. (1989). *Frameworks of power*. Sage.

Collier, A. (1994). *An introduction to Roy Bhaskar's philosophy*. Verso.

Danermark, B., Ekstrom, L., Jakobsen, L., & Karlsson, J. C. (2002). *Explaining society: Critical realism and the social sciences*. Routledge.

Davies, J. S., & Trounstine, J. (2012). Urban politics and the new institutionalism. In K. Mossberger, S. E. Clark, & P. John (Eds.), *The Oxford handbook of new urban politics*. Oxford University Press.

De Leeuw, E. (2009). Evidence for healthy cities: Reflections on practice, method and theory. *Health Promotion International, 24*(suppl_1), i19–i36.

De Leeuw, E. (2012). Do healthy cities work? A logic of method for assessing impact and outcome of healthy cities. *Journal of Urban Health, 89*(2), 217–231.

De Leeuw, E. (2017). Engagement of sectors other than health in integrated health governance, policy, and action. *Annual Review of Public Health, 38*(1), 329–349.

de Leeuw, E., & Skovgaard, T. (2005). Utility-driven evidence for healthy cities: Problems with evidence generation and application. *Social Science & Medicine, 61*(6), 1331–1341.

Downward, P., Finch, J. H., & Ramsay, J. (2002). Critical realism, empirical methods and inference: A critical discussion. *Cambridge Journal of Economics, 26*(4), 481–500.

Flyvbjerg, B. (2001). *Making social science matter: Why social inquiry fails and how it can succeed again.* Cambridge University Press.

Gaventa, J. (2006). Finding the spaces for change: A power analysis. *IDS Bulletin, 37*(6), 23–33.

Hall, P. A., & Taylor, R. C. R. (1996). Political science and the three new institutionalisms. *Political Studies, 44*(5), 936.

Harris, P., Baum, F., Friel, S., Mackean, T., Schram, A., & Townsend, B. (2020). A glossary of theories for understanding power and policy for health equity. *Journal of Epidemiology and Community Health, 74*, 548–552.

Harris, P., Friel, S., & Wilson, A. (2015). 'Including health in systems responsible for urban planning': A realist policy analysis research programme. *British Medical Journal Open, 5*(7), e008822.

Harris, P., & Haigh, F. (2015). Including Health in Environmental Impact Assessments: Is an institutional approach useful for practice? *Impact Assessment and Project Appraisal, 33*(2), 135–141.

Harris, P., Haigh, F., Thornell, M., Molloy, L., & Sainsbury, P. (2014a). Housing, health and master planning: Rules of engagement. *Public Health, 128*(4), 354–359.

Harris, P., Sainsbury, P., & Kemp, L. (2014b). The fit between health impact assessment and public policy: Practice meets theory. *Social Science & Medicine, 108*, 46–53.

Harris, P. J., Kemp, L. A., & Sainsbury, P. (2012). The essential elements of health impact assessment and healthy public policy: A qualitative study of practitioner perspectives. *British Medical Journal Open, 2*(6), e001245.

Harvey, D. (1987). Reconsidering social theory: A debate. *Environment and Planning d: Society and Space, 5*(4), 367–434.

Healey, P. (2006). Transforming governance: Challenges of institutional adaptation and a new politics of space. *European Planning Studies, 14*(3), 299–320.

Healey, P., Cars, G., Madanipour, A., & De Magalhaes, C. (2002a). Transforming governance, institutionalist analysis and institutional capacity. In G. Cars, P. Healey, A. Madanipour, & C. De Magalhães (Eds.), *Urban governance, institutional capacity and social milieux* (pp. 20–42). Routledge.

Horton, R. (2017). Offline: Medicine and Marx. *Lancet, 390*, 20126.

Howlett, M., Ramesh, M., & Perl, A. (2009). *Studying public policy: Policy cycles and policy sub-systems* (3rd ed.). Oxford University Press.

Immergut, E. M. (1998). The theoretical core of the new institutionalism. *Politics & Society, 26*(1), 5–34.

Immergut, E. M. (2006). *Historical-institutionalism in political science and the problem of change* (pp. 237–259). Springer.

Jenkins-Smith, H., Nohrstedt, D., Weible, C., & Sabatier, P. (2014). The advocacy coalition framework: Foundations, evolution, and ongoing research. In P. Sabatier & C. Weible (Eds.), *Theories of the policy process*. Routledge.

Jessop, B. (1998). The rise of governance and the risks of failure: The case of economic development. *International Social Science Journal, 50*(155), 29–45.

Jones, B. D., & Baumgartner, F. R. (2012). From there to here: Punctuated equilibrium to the general punctuation thesis to a theory of government information processing. *Policy Studies Journal, 40*(1), 1–20.

Kay, A. (2005). A critique of the use of path dependency in policy studies. *Public Administration, 83*(3), 553–571.

Kjær, A. M. (2009). Governance and the urban bureaucracy. In J. S. Davies & D. L. Imbroscio (Eds.), *Theories of urban politics* (pp. 137–152). Sage.

Koch, P. (2013). Overestimating the shift from government to governance: Evidence from Swiss metropolitan areas. *Governance, 26*(3), 397–423.

Lawson, T. (2003). *Reorienting economics*. New York, Routledge.

Layder, D. (1998). *Sociological practice: Linking theory and social research*. Sage.

Lowndes, V. (2001). Rescuing Aunt Sally: Taking institutional theory seriously in urban politics. *Urban Studies, 38*(11), 1953–1971.

Lowndes, V. (2009). New institutionalism and urban politics. In Jonathan S Davies, David Imbroscio (Eds.), *Theories of Urban Politics*, 2, (pp. 91–105). Sage.

March, J. G., & Olsen, J. P. (1986). *Rediscovering institutions: The organizational basis of politics*. Simon and Schuster.

March, J. G., & Olsen, J. P. (1996). Institutional perspectives on political institutions. *Governance, 9*(3), 247–264.

Marsh, D. (2009). Keeping ideas in their place: In praise of thin constructivism. *Australian Journal of Political Science, 44*(4), 679–696.

McQueen, D., & Anderson, L. M. (2001). What counts as evidence: Issues and debates. In I. Rootman, M. Goodstadt, B. Hyndman, D. V. McQueen,

L. Potvin, J. Springett, E. Ziglio, et al. (Eds.), *Evaluation in health promotion. Principles and perspectives* (pp. 63–82. European Series: 63–81). WHO Regional Publications.

Medvetz, T., & Sallaz, J. J. (2018). *The Oxford handbook of Pierre Bourdieu.* Oxford University Press.

Mingers, J. (2014). *Systems thinking, critical realism and philosophy: A confluence of ideas.* Routledge.

Ollman, B. (2001). Critical realism in the light of Marx's process of abstraction. In J. Lopez & G. Potter (Eds.), *After postmodernism: An introduction to critical realism* (pp. 1–16). Athlone.

Outhwaite, W. (1987). *New philosophies of social science: Realism, hermeneutics and critical theory.* MacMillan.

Pawson, R., & Tilley, N. (1997). *Realistic evaluation.* Sage.

Pierre, J., & Peters, B. G. (2012). Urban governance. In Karen Mossberger, Susan E. Clarke, Peter John (Eds.), *The Oxford handbook of urban politics.* Oxford University Press.

Potter, G., & Lopez, P. (2001). After postmodernism: The new millennium. In J. Lopez & G. Potter (Eds.), *After postmodernism: An introduction to critical realism* (1–16). Athlone.

Pratt, A. C. (1995). Putting critical realism to work: The practical implications for geographical research. *Progress in Human Geography, 19*(1), 61–74.

Rein, M., & Schön, D. (1996). Frame-critical policy analysis and frame-reflective policy practice. *Knowledge and Policy, 9*(1), 85–104.

Rhodes, R. A. (2007). Understanding governance: Ten years on. *Organization Studies, 28*(8), 1243–1264.

Savage, V., & Yeh, P. (2019). Novelist Cormac McCarthy's tips on how to write a great science paper. *Nature, 574*(7778), 441.

Sayer, A. (1992). *Method in social science: A realist approach* (2nd ed.). Routledge.

Sayer, A. (1998). Abstraction: A realist interpretation. In M. Archer, R. Bhaskar, A. Collier, T. Lawson, & A. Norrie (Eds.), *Critical realism: Essential readings* (pp. 120–143). Routledge.

Sayer, A. (2000). *Realism and social science.* Sage.

Schaler, E. (2014). An assessment of the institutional analysis and development framework and introduction of the social-ecological systems framework. In P. W. Sabatier & M. Christopher (Eds.), *Theories of the policy process.* Westview Press.

Scott, A. J., & Storper, M. (2015). The nature of cities: The scope and limits of urban theory. *International Journal of Urban and Regional Research, 39*(1), 1–15.

Scott, W. R. (2005). *Institutions and organizations: Ideas and interests* (3rd ed.). Sage.

Stoker, G. (1998). Governance as theory: Five propositions. *International Social Science Journal*, 50(155), 17–28.

Stone, C. N. (2015). Power. In E.Mossberger, S. Clarke, & J. Peter (Eds.), *Oxford handbook of urban politics*. Oxford University Press.

Stones, R. (1996). *Sociological reasoning: Towards a past-modern sociology*. Macmillan Press Ltd.

Tsouros, A. D. (2017). *Healthy cities: A political project designed to change how cities understand and deal with health* (pp. 489–504). Springer.

Weible, C. M. (2014). Introducing the scope and focus of policy process research and theory. In P. W. Sabatier & M. Christopher (Eds.), *Theories of the policy process* (p. 1). Westview Press.

Weiss, C. H. (1999). The interface between evaluation and public policy. *Evaluation*, 5(4), 468–486.

Williams, S. J. (2003). Beyond meaning, discourse and the empirical world: Critical realist reflections on health. *Social Theory & Health*, 1, 42–71.

Yeung, H. W. C. (1997). Critical realism and realist research in human geography: A method or a philosophy in search of a method? *Progress in Human Geography*, 21(1), 51–74.

Zahariadis, N. (2014). Ambiguity and multiple streams. In P. Sabatier & C. Weible (Eds.), *Theories of the policy process* (pp. 25–58). Westview Press.

CHAPTER 4

The Steps in Critical Realist Analysis

What is theory? How can theory be used to inform research? Where does theory fit in the research enterprise? What theory or theories can be developed by research? Each of these questions, and others, about theory have bedevilled the scientific endeavour. Perhaps they will forever. A critical realist methodology has special consideration of the role and place of theory. I use this chapter to articulate that consideration as part of a systematic set of steps that are involved in critical realist research and analysis.

The philosophical and conceptual underpinnings were presented in the previous chapters. Here, I unpack what theory is and provide practical steps to incorporating theory into analysis. I provide links to the later sections of the book that demonstrate the steps in practice. The chapter finishes by suggesting the development of adaptive theory as a laudable goal for public health policy analysis.

'Bricolage' was suggested by one reviewer of the manuscript as an analogy for the type of approach presented in the book. I quite like the term as it describes choosing building blocks to construct analysis. My review of the literature on bricolage showed some caveats for a critical realist, however. Much of the bricolage literature is concerned with mixed methods and a pragmatic take on epistemology that emphasises methods over and above theory. My use of methods is not as eclectic, so is not

© The Author(s), under exclusive license to Springer Nature Switzerland AG 2022
P. Harris, *Illuminating Policy for Health*, Palgrave Studies in Public Health Policy Research,
https://doi.org/10.1007/978-3-031-13199-8_4

methods bricolage. My 'bricolage' use of theory, however, is eclectic. My theoretical bricolage also conforms to the mixed use of empiricism and theory suggested by the scholar whose work aims to situate Bricolage in scholarly inquiry (Kincheloe, 2011).

THEORY AND RESEARCH: TYPES AND USES

The place of theory is arguably at the centre of all debates about scientific method (Crotty, 1998). Writing about healthy cities for instance, De Leeuw (2009) argues that 'in most scientific fields' being explicit about theory as a 'frame of reference' (p. i22) is what makes research valid and reliable (De Leeuw, 2009).

But what is theory? Box 4.1 explains how critical realists categorise different types of theory and theoretical knowledge. I borrowed heavily from Andrew Sayer's excellent introductory books to realist research (Sayer, 1992, 2000).

Box 4.1: Types of theories

Meta-theories concern foundational assumptions and preconditions of science. Examples are critical realism, phenomenology, hermeneutics and positivism, each of which are metatheories building on different ontologies and epistemologies (Danermark et al., 2002). All research is informed at a meta-theoretical level (Crotty, 1998). Critical realism happens to make meta-theory explicit (Collier, 1994).

Normative theories express, examine and support various ideas on how things ought to be—what 'should' happen'—and tend to be based moral, political or ideological issues and interests (Danermark et al., 2002).

Descriptive theories claim to be able to describe and characterise more fundamental properties, structures, internal relations and mechanisms, thereby suggesting how we may interpret and explain different social phenomena. Sayer (1992) further distinguishes two types of descriptive theory. One is theory as *ordering frameworks* (or filing systems) which permit observational data, the meaning of which is taken to be unproblematic, to be used for predicting and explaining empirical events.

Another is theory as *conceptualisation*, which means conceptualising 'events, mechanisms and internal relations in a certain way, with the help of theories' (p. 120; Sayer, 1992). These conceptualisations produce explanatory theories. *Explanatory theories* are the product of these full descriptive

---

conceptualisations that follow the steps outlined in this chapter and book. Their purpose is providing a full explanation of reality and its underlying mechanisms, powers and structures.

The crucial fault line in types of theorising introduced in box 4.1 is that between description for ordering purposes and conceptualisation for explanation (Sayer, 2000). The former will be familiar to many research approaches that either categorise empirical data by testing a hypothesis (positivistic deductivism) or constructing theories based solely on experiential data (constructivist inductivism). Explanatory theorising brings theory, in the manner of 'bricolage', to better explain that descriptive data.

At this juncture, it is useful to reflect on what the 'critical' in critical realism means. At its most basic, being 'critical', using theory, provides a check on reality such that analysis is more than the pragmatic representation of data. Considering health equity, for instance, description of the problem, usually through 'what questions', is not enough. Rather, against theory we can deepen explanations to ask 'how' and 'why' questions. Specific public health policy questions, for instance, include: Why are actors interested in health or not? Why do structures support health focussed policy? How do processes and decisions enable or block health ideas or strategies? How does governance foster healthy policymaking? How is power an obstacle or opportunity for a health focus? How has policy or policymaking created the inequities that are being experienced? Or, if interventions are the focus, why did the intervention improve health equity or not?

At the same time, linking back to theory situates (similarly to positivism) in knowledge that has gone before. Applying insights from a set of data a body of theory adds to the cumulative knowledge base. Using a crude analogy, theory, used critically, breaks us out of the hamster wheel of experience.

That said, theory needs to speak to the data with a clear and transparent position on what is being drawn out and why. My interests, for example, revolve understanding and explaining healthy public policy for health equity. Uncritical use of theory must be avoided, as I demonstrate in part 2 of the book by showing how particular urban political theorists have normative positions informing their theories with profound consequences for policymaking. History is replete with the misapplication of theory or knowledge for the sake of power and domination. Critical thinking about theory itself matters, especially when doing critical realist research. For instance, I recently reviewed a manuscript that argued, using Bhaskar, how critical realism allows access to the hitherto unseen hand of God (see Pawson, 2013, for a typically ascerbic take down of that element of Bhaskar's later work).

The realist evaluators Pawson and Tilley (1997) highlight that people do not know the full extent to which their world and behaviours are already being influenced. Theory and theorising, they argue, are therefore necessary to unpack what those influences are. Critical social science is similar, arguing that without a critical check scientific description merely reproduces reality regardless of how harmful that reality may be (Crotty, 1998). Public health researchers ought to be particularly attentive to an uncritical stance to our data. After all the main tenet of our discipline is 'do no harm'.

THE STEPS

One of the early misreadings of critical realism was that it is a philosophy without a method. This is not the case. I adapted the stages presented here from those outlined by Danermark et al. (2002) and Bhaskar. Bhaskar (see Box 4.2) developed a four-stage pattern of explanation in critical realist research investigating 'complex causal sequences' (p. 122) which he termed RRRE (Collier, 1994).

Box 4.2: Bhaskar's realist analysis steps.

- Resolution—the process is analysed into its various causal components
- re-description—granted that we have a background of theory about the various mechanisms operative in this open system, we can re-describe the causal components in terms of this theory. We will then be in a position to
- retroduct the causes of these components. However, since we are in an open system, there may be any number of possible causes that could have co-determined these events. We need to

---

- eliminate such of these as we can, by means of independent evidence about the antecedent events.

In Table 4.1, I present the systematic stepwise approach to undertaking realist informed policy analysis or research. Other critical realist authors emphasise similar stages. For example, Outhwaite (1987) provides three rules of thumb for understanding complex open systems (Outhwaite, 1987). The first is theoretical abstraction, since 'observational' statements have no special privilege. The second is to fit particular explanations within a wider context that governs the structures and mechanisms of reality. The third requires connecting 'a priori' theories with these developed explanatory propositions. For instance, Outhwaite's first two stages are enabled by situating data about policy against, the essential constructs presented at the end of Chapter 3. The third stage requires going back to a priori theory to then build explanatory propositions about what is really going on. This is shown in the 'application of theory' column in Table 4.1.

Note that most of the chapter numbers in Table 4.1 point you to Part 2 of the book where the practical application of the step is detailed. Below I detail the essentials in each step.

The first 'description' stage, just as the name suggests, describes the event one intends to study. For my research, this is healthy public policy and the relations this embodies. Emphasising the empirical world, Danermark et al. (2002) point out how description utilises 'everyday concepts... the interpretations of the persons involved and their way of describing the current situation' (p. 109). Experiential empirical data in other words. I use an a priori theory for this stage, given the object of my attention is healthy public policy. As detailed in previous chapters, healthy public policy is essentially concerned with institutions which can be empirically described by focussing on the dimensions of the policy cube.

The second stage, 'analytic resolution', is where the task of abstraction begins. I detailed abstraction in the previous chapter. The analysis begins to differentiate causal mechanisms and structures by separating 'concrete' objects into various components, aspects or dimensions (Bhaskar, 1978; Sayer, 1998). At the same time, one of the purposes of this stage is a narrowing one given that reality [especially of policy] is complex. Choosing what to cover is vital.

Table 4.1 Theoretical Bricolage approach to policy analysis and research

Step	What happens	Application of theory	Chapter example
Description	Empirically describe phenomena and events	Data collection using policy cube as a priori framework	5, 7
Analytic resolution	Work out dimensions of phenomena and isolate what to investigate	Detailed analysis of data against SIAP (structures, ideas, actors, processes) or policy cube categories (see Chapter 5), potentially including 'context'	5, 7
Comparison between different theories	Reject some theories in favour of others more appropriate for the research	Review bodies of theory against core empirical findings (e.g. theories of the policy process, governance, power, urban politics, sociology)	8
Abduction/retroduction	Redescribe events of interest, based on theoretical concepts / use theory to explain mechanisms and structures	Apply new theoretically informed knowledge to redescribe the data/shift attention to underlying causal mechanisms and influencing conditions	9–10
Concretisation and contextualisation	Return to data to confirm theoretical redescription with real-world data	Reapply or test theoretical problems to the original data or collect new data	9–10

I brought the third stage, theoretical comparison, forward from where Danermark et al. (2002) position it. This systematic comparison of theories against the data has a goal of retaining theories that speak to the data and those that do not. As I later detail, I usually begin with compendiums of particular areas of theory. Trial runs usually only take a few minutes before the connections are clear. Muddier connections take longer. Going down the wrong theoretical path usually becomes quickly apparent. Quickly reject those theories that have limited connection to the data for those that do.

The fourth stage of the analysis intertwines what Danermark et al. (2002) separate out as 'abduction and theoretical redescription' and 'retroduction'.[1] 'Abduction/theoretical redescription' connects data to theory. This use of theory provides the possibility of thinking more confidently about the causal relations between objects detailed in Chapter 3. However, confidence is difficult without also including the analysis described in the retroduction stage. Retroduction explains the mechanisms and structures, in the light of theory, which are characteristic and constitutive of the structures of the object of investigation. Importantly in terms of sources of theory for retroduction, I tend to go deeper into the body of knowledge initially identified in the previous step which focusses on comparing theories. Going deeper means reading more literature and often particular bodies of theory. This can be time consuming but is vital. The end point of retroduction is to develop propositions that fully explain the empirical data critically and with depth.

Danermark, Ekstrom et al. suggest a sixth stage, 'concretisation and contextualisation' (similar to Bhaskar's final 'elimination' stage in RRRE in box 4.1). This step situates how the identified objects and relations between them manifest themselves in concrete reality, under specific conditions. There are two ways of approaching this stage. One is to collect more data that affirm or disconfirm the causal analysis. The other option is to return to the original data and work through it. Often deeper causal analysis of that original data alerts you to other pieces of data that had been previously missed but that hold firm against the causal propositions developed in retroduction.

---

[1] Notably Bhaskar (1978) focusses on retroduction in the third stage of the RRRE.

THE GOAL: ADAPTIVE THEORY

Comprehensive analysis needs a goal to be useful for knowledge and practice. 'Adaptive theory' covers many of the attributes of such a goal. Adaptive theory is the construction of novel theory that utilises both prior theory and theory that emerges from data collection and analysis. Adaptive theory offers a 'theoretical scaffold' (Layder, 1998; p. 150) which is relatively durable because it adapts (hence the name) reflexively with empirical data. Further, adaptability means the ability to reconfigure to accommodate new information. Adaptive theory draws on the elements of both Grounded Theory (Glaser & Strauss, 1967) and middle range theory (Merton, 1967). Both these approaches stress the importance of the relationship between empirical research and the development of theory as a precondition for the cumulative growth of (sociological) knowledge (Layder, 1998).

CONCLUSION

This chapter provided a tentative practical framework for healthy public policy research. The use of theory to explain empirical data lies at the heart of the framework. To that end, I borrowed heavily throughout from the articulation of what theory is and how to systematically incorporate theory into a research enterprise that has a goal of explaining, critically, what is going on in reality. I concluded by introducing adaptive theory as a goal for the comprehensive analysis the chapter advocates.

REFERENCES

Bhaskar, R. (1978). *A Realist theory of science* (3rd ed.). Verso.

Collier, A. (1994). *An introduction to Roy Bhaskar's philosophy*. Verso.

Crotty, M. (1998). *The foundations of social research: Meaning and perspective in the research process*. Sage.

Danermark, B., Ekstrom, L., Jakobsen, L., & Karlsson, J. C. (2002). *Explaining society: Critical realism and the social sciences*. Routledge.

De Leeuw, E. (2009). Evidence for healthy cities: reflections on practice, method and theory. Health promotion international *24*(suppl. 1), i19–i36.

Glaser, B., & Strauss, A. (1967). *The discovery of grounded theory*. Aldine.

Kincheloe, J. L. (2011). On to the next level: Continuing the conceptualization of the bricolage. *Key works in critical pedagogy* (pp. 253–277), Brill.

Layder, D. (1998). *Sociological practice: Linking theory and social research.* Sage Publications.

Merton, R. (1967). *On theoretical sociology.* Free Press.

Outhwaite, W. (1987). *New philosophies of social science: Realism, hermeneutics and critical theory.* MacMillan.

Pawson, R. (2013). *The science of evaluation: A realist manifesto.* Sage.

Pawson, R., & Tilley, N. (1997). *Realistic evaluation.* Sage.

Sayer, A. (1992). *Method in social science: A realist approach* (2nd ed.). Routledge.

Sayer, A. (1998). Abstraction: A realist interpretation. In M. Archer, R. Bhaskar, A. Collier, T. Lawson, & A. Norrie (Eds.), *Critical realism: Essential readings* (pp. 120–143). Routledge.

Sayer, A. (2000). *Realism and social science.* Sage Publications.

CHAPTER 5

Drawing Out the Essentials for Analysing Public Policy for Health

In all honesty, I struggled to fit this chapter at this point of the book. I initially had included this at the end of Chapter 3. That was because the categories outlined provide the roadmap for analysing policy with the floodlights on. The chapter fits better here, however, covering as it does the first two stages in the critical realist analytic steps introduced last chapter, 'description' and 'analytic resolution'. At the same time, it acts as a bridge to shift focus from critical realism onto policy. Policy is, after all, the book's object of attention. The concepts presented provide 'a priori' categories to break up the essential elements of policy. Boldly, I claim here that they are the essentials of policy that, on my review at least, are found across the literature. As a framework of universal descriptors, they provide the basis for data collection and initial analysis about a particular policy under scrutiny (how to do this is the focus of the next two chapters at the start of part 2).

I also confess to cheating a bit in the presentation of the framework. The absolute core, what I call 'structures, actors, ideas and processes', came about through my reading and reviewing the policy literature. The other categories came about by me doing research about policy. Power and governance in particular came in later as I was doing the research detailed in part 2 of the book. In this way, then, the framework is a bit a priori (coming before the research) and a bit a posteriori (after the

© The Author(s), under exclusive license to Springer Nature Switzerland AG 2022
P. Harris, *Illuminating Policy for Health*, Palgrave Studies in Public Health Policy Research,
https://doi.org/10.1007/978-3-031-13199-8_5

research). That iterative approach, however, is part of the critical realist approach (Danermark et al., 2002; Sayer, 1998, 2000).

Before entering into the detail, I need to make a disclaimer about the contents of the bottle. The purpose of this series this book belongs to is to connect public health and political science research. I do that in part, but not fully. Nor would I claim to. My effort with the book as a whole, and this section in particular, is to provide a roadmap for public health policy/healthy public policy analysis. As I noted in the introduction chapter, I cannot do justice to the whole library of knowledge from disciplines such as political science. Rather, here I use my critical realist lens, largely focussed on drawing out differences between structure and agency, to navigate what it is about policy, and policy institutions that can be the basis for a detailed analysis of real-world instances of healthy public policy. Thankfully, I am not alone in such attempts. Patrick Fafard, Evelyne De Leeuw (Editors of this book series) and others have similarly used theory to unpack 'health political science' (Fafard et al., 2021). My work is in the same vein as them—to better understand public policy to better influence health and health equity. Of note, however, is that political scientists have also presented similar frameworks to unpack the essentials of policy (Cairney et al., 2019). The notably difference between our efforts is that their object of attention is the complexities of policy, whereas mine is how health is considered in public policy.

My entry point to the essential elements is the excellent introductory text to political science tellingly titled, 'Policy Cycles and Subsystems' (Howlett et al., 2009). For health professionals or those new to policy, that text book, and its later editions (Howlett et al., 2020), usefully documents a history of policy studies and political science. They introduce their analysis as in the tradition of new institutionalism and in particular a 'statist' (emphasising the role of the state) variant to that institutionalist body of public policy knowledge. Statism, interestingly, links back to critical realist takes on public policy, especially the work of authors like Bob Jessop that has morphed into sophisticated theorising and research about governance and power (Jessop, 2001, 2005, 2007). I return to similar thinking in detail in part 2. For now, though, my focus is on the core dynamics of policy provided by statism, which uses an institutional lens. Again, I caution that this is my take on new institutionalism for the purposes of this book and my analysis. New institutionalism is a body of work that has a much longer history and depth than that which I provide here. This is my walk through the library where I have picked the concepts that I find provide the core for analytically breaking down what the essentials of policy are.

New Institutionalism: A Brief History

New institutionalism broadly focusses attention on the dynamics of policy institutions to unpack how public policy is made and under what conditions (Immergut, 1998; Cairney, 2011; Harris et al., 2015). Analytically, four—initially three—types of 'new institutionalism' help articulate the essentials of what matters for turning the floodlights on healthy public policy (for a more detailed history, see (Peters, 2019): rational choice, historical, sociological and most recently discursive (Hall & Taylor, 1996, Lowndes, 2001). Each was developed independently from each other, but similarly as a reaction to the behavioural perspectives dominant in political science from the 1950s (Immergut, 1998). In the urban politics literature, Lowndes has provided perhaps the best overviews of the differences (Lowndes, 2001, 2009). I've also recently written about these differences by centring in on power and health equity in policy (Harris et al., 2020).

As floodlights, new institutionalist thinking focusses attention on fundamentals of policy systems: structure, agency and ideas (Marsh, 2009). Rational choice approaches emphasise agency. Sociological and historical approaches defer to structures—culture and organisation in the former, historically determined social constructions in the latter. Discursive mixes agency with ideas and structures.

The big schism across all of them is whether they allow an analysis of change (Immergut, 2006). Essentially, for something to be institutionalised—like healthy public policy or health equity in policy decision-making—an institution must change to take on that idea, and analysis must attend to processes and structures that led to that outcome occurring or not (Healey, 2006; De Leeuw, 2009). Big structural theories like Marxism struggle to describe local possibilities or actions that are change focussed. Agentic, often behavioural, approaches struggle to have a wide enough lens on context, culture and time. This tension between agency and structure is not new and lies at the heart of most if not all philosophising about society and power (Flyvbjerg, 2001, Harris et al., 2020). What is needed, of course, is a balance between the two that draws out what is happening in the empirical data to then provide a deeper explanation in terms of both stasis and change. If you would like to go deeper into arguments about structure and agency, I suggest reading both Sayer (2000) and Archer (1995) in the critical realism literature. Pierre Bourdieu takes strongly similar positions in the sociology literature (Medvetz & Sallaz, 2018).

ESSENTIALISING PUBLIC [HEALTH]
POLICY: THE POLICY CUBE

Here, I present the essential factors, or 'units of analysis', that are the bedrock of this book[1]. Given the 'urban' policy focus of this book, I've sprinkled in some flavouring from the urban literature (Fig. 5.1).

To the left, I use 'Institutions' as the descriptor that covers the three core dimensions of policy: structures, ideas and actors.

'*Structures*' are overt or implicit (often unrecognised) social and institutional, macro-societal, conditions that act as the famous 'rules of the game' in terms of expectations about how the game should be played and who has power in the game (Arts & Van Tatenhove, 2004). Structures have several dimensions including rules and lines of command, divisions of labour, resources, responsibility and channels of communication (Howlett et al., 2009). These institutional structures provide the conditions (Schaler, 2014) controlling how or why health may be incorporated or not across the urban and regional planning system, as well as how the health sector engages with that system. Structures are operationalised through the rules and mandates that influence lines of command, divisions of labour, resources, responsibility and channels of communication (Fuchs & Lederer, 2007). Structuralist approaches emphasise overt or implicit (often unrecognised) social and institutional, macro-societal, conditions that influence policy decisions and choices (Arts & Van Tatenhove, 2004).

---

[1] There are variants across the political science literature, for instance 'Ideas, institutions and interests' Weiss, C. H. (1999). "The interface between evaluation and public policy." Evaluation 5(4): 468–486, Peters, B. G. (2019). Institutional theory in political science: The new institutionalism, Edward Elgar Publishing. But I feel actors, ideas, structures's differentiation is able to better tease apart the critical realist emphasis on differentiating structure and agency. Others have emphasised 'context' as surrounding policy but not necessarily able to be influenced. I have instead folded context into the analysis, because context may in fact be influential and in turn be influenced and thus is not, according to critical realists, 'independent' from the other factors in the policy cube (indeed it is constituted by them). Cairney et al. add 'events' as external influences on policy (following Sabatier and others), but here I focus on them as outcomes from policy decisions. There is I think more work to be done on these essential characteristics. I present here, using a realist lens, is necessary and essential factors. Other concepts, like interests and institutions, may be what critical realists call 'mechanisms' that fire up those essentials. However, and with a pragmatic hat on, while this conceptualising about policy is of course interesting, in the end it may not actually matter that much given the similarities between factors.

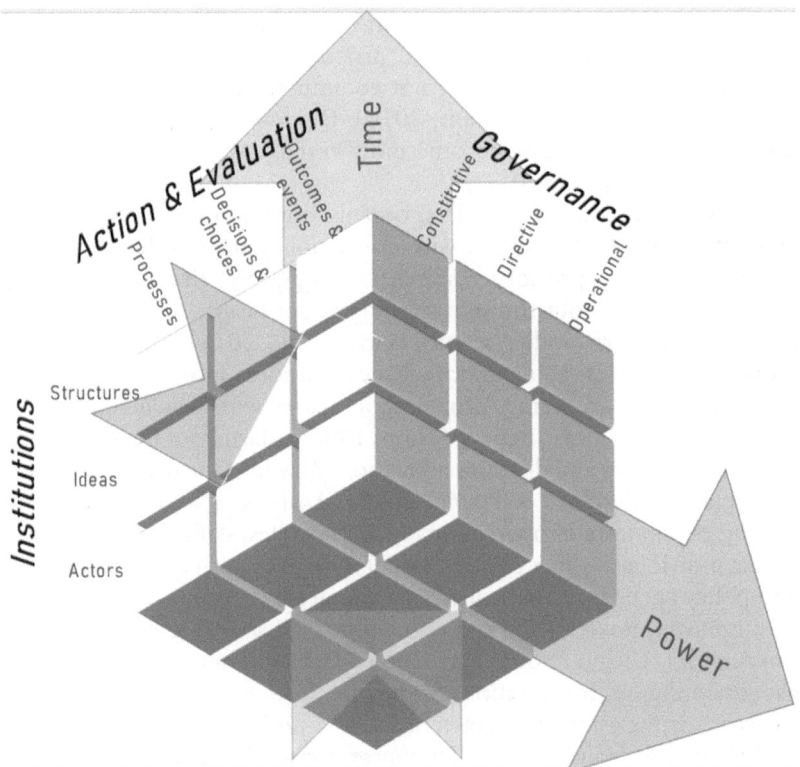

Fig. 5.1 (Healthy) public policy cube

Ideas refer to the content of issues in policies, plans and procedures. For health as a cross-sectoral public policy issue, there remain definitional tensions—does it refer to 'hospitals', 'illness', 'wellbeing' or 'equity'? (Harris et al., 2014). For the business of another sector, the idea of health needs to connect to the substantive issues driving that sector (Harris et al., 2016), for example the importance of economic development and/or environmental sustainability for urban and regional planning. I tend to include the role of evidence and data in planning here. Concerning ideas, discourse matters. Discourse covers a mix of norms, ideas and societal institutions that reflect and become part of communicative practices and cultural values (Fuchs & Lederer, 2007). Discourse is thus the term used to capture the substantive content of ideas—'core beliefs' (Sabatier, 1988)—as well as the practices and processes through which ideas are conveyed and communicated (or not communicated) in institutions and by actors (Carstensen & Schmidt, 2016). Discourse is the point in policy in which political contests become most visible and values and interests made clearest (Cairney, 2011).

Actors include the stakeholders, organisations and networks (Jenkins-Smith et al., 2014). Consistent with classic policy analysis theory (Hall & Taylor, 1996), my previous research has suggested that policy change principally comes about through learning about health as a relevant issue for the business of another sector (Harris et al., 2014). Different policy actors bring 'frames' about specific issues and ideas into the policy arena which, like a picture frame, provide boundaries with which actors value and position their ideas (Rein & Schön, 1996). Mastery of the frames that define policy issues and domains allows for entry into the discourse of new policy players (Bilodeau & Potvin, 2018). Analysis of actors includes the opening of windows of opportunity based on roles, skills and strategies of specific individuals—policy entrepreneurs—in progressing ideas and issues onto policy agendas (Zahariadis, 2014). Crucially, *'Actors'* are also collectives: industry, government and regulators, civil society groups and local communities (Clegg, 1989; Scott, 2005). Indeed, I am often of the mind that separating out organisations from individuals is a useful strategy when the search is for essential characteristics of a policy system (Harris et al., 2014; Harris & Haigh, 2015). Discourse is crucial once again and introduces a way of describing discursive communities, called 'hegemonies'. 'Hegemonies' (Howarth, 2010) form among actors who share resources and interpretations of a policy discourse, identify (more or less) similar policy goals and engage in policy processes to achieve those goals (Arts & Van Tatenhove, 2004). Hegemonies are both political practices—emphasising actors' values and interests that capture the making and breaking of coalitions—and ways of winning over consent or securing compliance via negotiation and bargaining to either reproduce or challenge established structures and discourses (Howarth, 2010).

Across the top of the cube is 'action and evaluation'.

'Processes' are first. *'Processes'* cover ways of working in policy systems, or 'how we go about things around here'. Processes are conditioned by the institutional dynamics of policy subsystems. These might be informal, as in the ways meetings are set or work is commissioned (such as a preference for in-house analysis or bringing in external advice) or

more formal policy procedures (e.g. regulations, expert advice, specifically commissioned studies, community consultations, checklists). In the policy literature, emphasis is placed on 'Procedures' (Howlett, et al., 2009). My previous research has shown how procedures became important mechanisms for including health in urban policymaking, for example expert advice, specifically commissioned studies, community consultations, checklists and types of impact assessments (Harris et al., 2014).

I then added 'decisions and choices' and then 'outcomes and events' as next in the causal chain of action and evaluation. Crucially, and perhaps surprising to a public health researcher, political scientists (Cairney, 2011) and Urban Political scholars (Stone, 2015) are clear that evaluating outcomes is extremely challenging given the timeframes and causal complexities from a policy to a measurable change like a health outcome. They suggest that 'directions' (Stone, 2015) or 'choices' (Cairney, 2011) are the main impacts that can be measured. 'Policy choices' concern decisions that are made by actors and that either perpetuate or challenge the institutional status quo (Cairney, 2011). Choice is important in policy because it brings in agency and decision-making as the fundamental 'outcome' of policymaking that can, sometimes at least, be observed. In the urban politics literature, when writing about power (see below), Clarence Stone (2015) makes some important observations about research focussing on Policy Directions as the equivalent to 'outcomes'. Directions are observable, Stone argues, whereas 'outcomes' are in many cases too far removed from policy action and systems to be observable. In my view, likely because of my public health training, outcomes are something to strive to evaluate. That said, I prefer borrowing the concept of (observable) 'events' from Sayer (1992).[2]

To the right is Governance.

Governance is literally everywhere in public policy, both as an idea and as an actual thing. As an idea governance is now extremely popular, capturing the zeitgeist of not only policymaking but (post) modern society. As an actual thing, it is, however, difficult to define and therefore apply. At its essence, governance is about networks of stakeholders involved in policymaking that include but go beyond government (Jessop,

---

[2] Sayer (1992; p 213) provides a schematic that most clearly represents the analytic process involved in critical research analysis. Notably that initial framework was extended by Margaret Archer (1995) to be core to her analytic approach. Archer comes back into the analysis later in the book.

1998; Stoker, 1998; Rhodes, 2007). Multi-level governance to progress health in public health policy requires action at multiple institutional levels: constitutive (i.e. designing institutions and norms); directive (i.e. rule setting and application); and operational (i.e. management of stakeholders and processes) (De Leeuw, 2017). Urbanists have provided some excellent and deep analyses of governance that I return to in part 2 (Healey, 2006; Kjaer, 2009; Pierre & Peters, 2012). As noted already, the scholar Bob Jessop—a critical realist, urbanist, governance and State power expert—has written one of the best introductory articles on governance as a dynamic mix of factors (Jessop, 1998).

Power is crucial to institutions. Power has been described as the most important factor for urban research (Clarke, 2015). Power, I noted earlier, has been somewhat of a touchstone in terms of where new institutionalism takes off from older political science theory. New institutionalism has tended to underplay power explicitly, perhaps because the exercise of power by individuals was the core mechanism in early behaviouralist approaches to policy. One of my tasks over the life of the research I report in Part 2 of this book was better understanding power for its use in policy analysis. After numerous attempts, I realised why I had struggled and what to do about this (Harris et al., 2020). Power is core to institutions and any type of policy analysis. But power is operationalised by structures, actors and their ideas. What comes through much of the political (urban and political science) literature is that there is a normative swing between seeing power as something that is wielded by individuals to effect change—often through an empowerment lens—or as 'structuring' the beliefs and actions of individuals. Analysis requires both, depending of course on actual experiences, cases or data under scrutiny.

The concept of the policy cube was inspired by the Power Cube (Gaventa, 2006). Gaventa was himself inspired many prior ideas about power, which he turned into a multi-level cube. Power as represented by the power cube crosses levels from local to global (levels of power), is more or less open to influence and can be closed off or opened up (spaces of power), and is often invisible or hidden even while being ever present (visibility of power). Connected to the analysis presented in this book, colleagues and I have produced a complementary but much more comprehensive analysis of power across levels and 'venues' of public health policymaking (Friel et al., 2021).

Time is the final critical unit shaping policy systems. The long-term tendency in policy is towards 'path dependency' which is institutionalised way of making policy that are hard, if not impossible, to shift (Kay, 2005; Koch, 2013). The reasons are institutional and bring us back to the dynamics presented in the cube. For instance, urban focussed research has shown how new policy ideas and new governance approaches face an uphill battle challenging existing urban policy power structures and dynamics (Healey et al., 2002; Scott & Storper, 2015). Changes, however, can and do happen however, often in quite sudden 'punctuations', when the mix of factors across the cube come together (Kay, 2005; Jones & Baumgartner, 2012).

CONCLUSION

Critical realist policy research is helped by an anchoring set of 'essential' parameters to policies under scrutiny. To that end, this chapter took a critical realist lens to the political science literature to arrive at the core attributes of policy institutions involved in public health policy. I presented those attributes in the form of a cube. The categories in the cube subsequently become the entry point to the data collection and analysis I present in the second half of the book.

A final note to this chapter is to repeat that my intent is for a public health policy audience. Each of the dynamics presented in this chapter comes together to lay the foundations for comprehensive, floodlit, analyses of public health policy in practice. Health is, as explained in Chapter 2, political, and the influence of policy on health occurs through a mix of structural, agentic and ideational factors. Indeed, these types of constructs have been recently empirically validated as essential for building health focussed evaluation capacity (Schwarzman et al., 2021)! Further, in terms of action and evaluation, how policymaking influences health is well known, and well validated, in evaluation circles to be a mix of process, impact and outcome factors. Here, I have added nuance from critical realism and other policy-related fields to focus attention on decisions and events.

Governance and power bring in additional depth and nuance to policy analysis. A critical realist analysis of policy necessitates the search for deeper explanations about structural influences on [the health] of society, the importance of agency, how power flows across both, as well as attending to institutions, governance, processes, decisions and outcomes.

The policy cube presented here provides the basic dimensions of that deeper analysis.

As a final caution in a chapter full of cautionary notes, this figure is an heuristic to collect and then analyse data against. Reality is much much more messy.

REFERENCES

Archer, M. S. (1995). *Realist social theory: The morphogenetic approach.* Cambridge University Press.

Arts, B., & Van Tatenhove J. (2004). Policy and power: A conceptual framework between the 'old'and 'new' policy idioms. *Policy Sciences, 37*(3–4): 339–356.

Bilodeau, A., & Potvin, L. (2018). Unpacking complexity in public health interventions with the actor-network theory. *Health Promotion International, 33*(1), 173–181.

Bhaskar, R. (1978). *A realist theory of science* (3rd ed.). Verso.

Cairney, P. (2011). *Understanding public policy: Theories and issues.* Palgrave Macmillan.

Cairney, P., Heikkila, T., & Wood, M. (2019). *Making policy in a complex world.* Cambridge University Press.

Carstensen, M. B., & Schmidt, V. A. (2016). Power through, over and in ideas: Conceptualizing ideational power in discursive institutionalism. *Journal of European Public Policy, 23*(3), 318–337.

Clarke, S. E. (2015). Emerging research agendas. In K. Mossberger, S. E. Clarke, & P. John (Eds.), *The Oxford handbook of urban politics.*

Clegg, S. R. (1989). *Frameworks of power.* Sage.

Collier, A. (1994). *An introduction to Roy Bhaskar's philosophy.* Verso.

Crotty, M. (1998). *The foundations of social research: Meaning and perspective in the research process.* Sage.

Danermark, B., Ekstrom, L., Jakobsen, L., & Karlsson, J. C. (2002). *Explaining society: Critical realism and the social sciences.* Routledge.

De Leeuw, E. (2009). Evidence for healthy cities: Reflections on practice, method and theory. *Health Promotion International, 24*(suppl. 1), i19–i36.

De Leeuw, E. (2017). Engagement of sectors other than health in integrated health governance, policy, and action. *Annual Review of Public Health, 38*(1), 329–349.

Fafard, P., Cassola, A., & de Leeuw, E. (2021). *Public health political science: Integrating science and politics for public health.* Springer.

Flyvbjerg, B. (2001). *Making social science matter: Why social inquiry fails and how it can succeed again.* Cambridge University Press.

Friel, S., Townsend, B., Fisher, M., Harris, P., Freeman, T., Baum, F. J. (2021, August). Power and the people's health. *Social Science and Medicine, 282,* 114173.

Fuchs, D., & Lederer, M. M. (2007). The power of business. *Business and Politics, 9*(3), 1–17.

Gaventa, J. (2006). Finding the spaces for change: A power analysis. *IDS Bulletin, 37*(6), 23–33.

Glaser, B., & Strauss, A. (1967). *The discovery of grounded theory.* Aldine.

Harris, P., Friel, S., & Wilson, A. (2015). 'Including health in systems responsible for urban planning': A realist policy analysis research programme. *British Medical Journal Open, 5*(7), e008822.

Harris, P., & Haigh, F. (2015). Including health in environmental impact assessments: Is an institutional approach useful for practice? *Impact Assessment and Project Appraisal, 33*(2), 135–141.

Harris, P., Kent, J., Sainsbury, P., & Thow, A.-M. (2016). Framing health for land-use planning legislation: A qualitative descriptive content analysis. *Social Science & Medicine, 148,* 42–51.

Harris, P., Sainsbury, P., & Kemp, L. (2014). The fit between health impact assessment and public policy: Practice meets theory. *Social Science & Medicine, 108,* 46–53.

Harris, P., Baum, F., Friel, S., Mackean, T., Schram, A., & Townsend, B. (2020). A glossary of theories for understanding power and policy for health equity. *Journal of Epidemiology and Community Health, 74,* 548–552.

Healey, P. (2006). Transforming governance: Challenges of institutional adaptation and a new politics of space. *European Planning Studies, 14*(3): 299–320.

Healey, P., Cars, G., Madanipour, A., & de Magalhães, C. (2002b). Urban governance capacity in complex societies: challenges of institutional adaptation. In G. Cars, P. Healey, A., Madanipour, & C. De Magalhães (Eds.), *Urban governance, institutional capacity and social milieux* (pp. 204–225).

Howarth, D. (2010). Power, discourse, and policy: Articulating a hegemony approach to critical policy studies. *Critical Policy Studies, 3*(3–4), 309–335.

Howlett, M., Ramesh, M., & Perl, A. (2009). *Studying public policy: Policy cycles and policy sub-systems* (3rd ed.). Oxford University Press.

Howlett, M., Ramesh, M., & Perl, A. (2020). *Studying public policy: Principles and processes.* Oxford University Press.

Immergut, E. M. (1998). The theoretical core of the new institutionalism. *Politics & Society, 26*(1), 5–34.

Immergut, E. M. (2006). Historical-institutionalism in political science and the problem of change. In *Understanding Change* (pp. 237–259). Springer.

Jenkins-Smith, H., Nohrstedt, D., Weible, C., & Sabatier, P. (2014). The advocacy coalition framework: Foundations, evolution, and ongoing research. In P. Sabatier & C. Weible (Eds.), *Theories of the policy process*. Routledge.

Jessop, B. (1998). The rise of governance and the risks of failure: The case of economic development. *International Social Science Journal, 50*(155), 29–45.

Jessop, B. (2001). Institutional re(turns) and the strategic—Relational approach. *33*(7): 1213–1235.

Jessop, B. (2005). Critical realism and the strategic-relational approach. *New Formations, 56*(1), 40–53.

Jessop, B. (2007). *State power*. Polity.

Jones, B. D., & Baumgartner, F. R. (2012). From there to here: Punctuated equilibrium to the general punctuation thesis to a theory of government information processing. *Policy Studies Journal, 40*(1), 1–20.

Kay, A. (2005). A critique of the use of path dependency in policy studies. *Public Administration, 83*(3), 553–571.

Kjær, A. M. (2009). Governance and the urban bureaucracy. In J. S. Davies & D. L. Imbroscio (Eds.), *Theories of urban politics* (pp. 137–152). Sage.

Koch, P. (2013). Overestimating the shift from government to governance: Evidence from Swiss metropolitan areas. *Governance, 26*(3), 397–423.

Layder, D. (1998). *Sociological practice: Linking theory and social research*. Sage Publications.

Lowndes, V. (2001). Rescuing Aunt Sally: Taking institutional theory seriously in urban politics. *Urban Studies, 38*(11), 1953–1971.

Lowndes, V. (2009). New institutionalism and urban politics. In J. Davies, & D. Imbroscio (Eds.), *Theories of urban politics*. 91–105.

Marsh, D. (2009). Keeping ideas in their place: In praise of thin constructivism. *Australian Journal of Political Science, 44*(4), 679–696.

Medvetz, T., & Sallaz J. J. (2018). *The Oxford handbook of Pierre Bourdieu*. Oxford University Press.

Merton, R. (1967). *On theoretical sociology*. Free Press.

Outhwaite, W. (1987). *New philosophies of social science: Realism, hermeneutics and critical theory*. MacMillan.

Pawson, R., & Tilley, N. (1997). *Realistic evaluation*. Sage Publications.

Peters, B. G. (2019). *Institutional theory in political science: The new institutionalism*. Edward Elgar Publishing.

Pierre, J., & Peters, B. G. (2012). Urban governance. In K. Mossberger, S. E. Clarke, & P. John (Eds.), *The Oxford handbook of urban politics*.

Rein, M., & Schön, D. (1996). Frame-critical policy analysis and frame-reflective policy practice. *Knowledge and Policy, 9*(1), 85–104.

Rhodes, R. A. (2007). Understanding governance: Ten years on. *Organization Studies, 28*(8), 1243–1264.

Sabatier, P. A. (1988). An advocacy coalition framework of policy change and the role of policy-oriented learning therein. *Policy Sciences, 21*(2), 129–168.

Sayer, A. (1992). *Method in social science: A realist approach* (2nd ed.). Routledge.

Sayer, A. (1998). Abstraction: A realist interpretation. In M. Archer, R. Bhaskar, A. Collier, T. Lawson, & A. Norrie (Eds.), *Critical realism: Essential readings* (pp. 120–143). Routledge.

Sayer, A. (2000). *Realism and social science*: Sage Publications.

Schaler, E. (2014). An assessment of the institutional analysis and development framework and introduction of the social-ecological systems framework. In P. Sabatier & C. Weible (Eds.), *Theories of the Policy Process* (p. 267). Westview.

Scott, W. R. (2005). *Institutions and Organizations: Ideas and Interests* (3rd ed.). Sage Publications.

Scott, A. J., & Storper, M. (2015). The nature of cities: The scope and limits of urban theory. *International Journal of Urban and Regional Research, 39*(1), 1–15.

Schwarzman, J., Bauman, A., Gabbe, B. J., Rissel, C., Shilton, T., Smith, B. J. J. E., & Planning, P. (2021). How practitioner, organisational and system-level factors act to influence health promotion evaluation capacity: Validation of a conceptual framework. *Evaluation and Program Planning, 91*, 102019.

Stoker, G. (1998). Governance as theory: Five propositions. *International Social Science Journal, 50*(155), 17–28.

Stone, C. N. (2015). Power. In E. Mossberger, S. Clarke, & J. Peter (Eds.), *Oxford handbook of urban politics*. Oxford University Press.

Zahariadis, N. (2014). Ambiguity and multiple streams. In P. Sabatier & C. Weible (Eds.), *Theories of the policy process* (pp. 25–58). Westview Press.

Section 1: Conducting a Realist Research Program into Health in Urban and Regional Planning in Australia, 2011–2021

This part of this book applies the methodology detailed in part I to a program of research on urban and regional planning in New South Wales (and South Australia), Australia. The first section covers the research protocol, empirical findings and the theories used. The second section applies those theories to provide deeper explanations about each of the case studies. I finish the book a set of recommendations to progress action on the findings of the research.

CHAPTER 6

Research Protocol

This chapter provides the protocol for the research presented in the rest of the book. The aim of the chapter is twofold. On the one hand, I present a robust research design for scrutiny. The protocol, by clearly articulating how the research proceeded, provides internal and external validity for the research. The initial presentation of the cases provides the backdrop to the more detailed development of the findings presented in subsequent chapters of this book. In particular, the protocol sets the scene behind each layer of the urban and regional planning system that is the object of investigation in the research program.

INTRODUCTION

This study investigates how, why and the extent to which health is considered in different functions of the policy system governing land-use planning in New South Wales (NSW), Australia. My focus was to interrogate the actual practice of the functions of that system. These functions are laid out in legislation and cover different layers of the land-use planning system in NSW (Harris et al., 2007). I was always bemused with the limited awareness among the public health sector of the regulatory, institutionalised, aspects of the planning system. So those workings were what I set about investigating.

© The Author(s), under exclusive license to Springer Nature Switzerland AG 2022
P. Harris, *Illuminating Policy for Health*, Palgrave Studies in Public Health Policy Research,
https://doi.org/10.1007/978-3-031-13199-8_6

The focus for the research was on three aspects of the system: legislation, strategic planning (often termed spatial planning in other contexts) and development assessments of very large infrastructure projects (in NSW called Environmental Assessments). Table 6.1 at the end of the chapter details the research program and includes relevant publications.

The entry point for the research was a novel opportunity to insert a 'health objective' during a reform process that happened between 2011 and 2013. This reform process stalled. However, it was possible to see the fruits of that 'health' focussed influence appear across the system in the years that followed. The research played out mostly in real time, though some of the case studies were based on documents referring to or reflections about plans and processes that had recently been completed. Planning as an enterprise (hence the name) occurs over long timeframes. Actual delivery comes about years after a plan or a project appraisal has been developed. The policy cycle is demonstrably mythical when applied to planning systems.

The failure of the reforms ostensibly closed the window for legislative influence. But a second, less public, process of reform went ahead. In 2018, new objectives were agreed—the overt 2013 health objective being replaced by one about 'place-based planning'. That 'place-based planning' objective was supported by a policy called 'Better Placed' (NSW Government Office of the Government Architect, 2018). That policy had 'health' as its primary goal.

Additionally, the activities which influenced the 2011–2013 review, particularly the inclusion of health, flowed through to other 'strategic' plans. The flow of health into those strategic activities is presented in Fig. 6.1. Almost immediately, the health advocacy in the 2011–2013 review influenced another major piece of land-use planning policy developed at the same time, the Sydney Metropolitan Strategy, first produced in 2013. That plan included health as one of four goals. A further set of plans were developed (produced in 2018) into a regional strategy and a further six metropolitan district plans. The final stage of the research focussed on the Western Sydney City Deal developed to integrate the strategic vision for a region with the delivery of infrastructure surrounding a second Sydney airport.

I also focussed on another side to any planning system, development assessment. This is the process by which particular developments are assessed for their impact before they are finally approved and then delivered. In many ways, these development assessments are the most

NSW Planning system activity and health's incremental inclusion

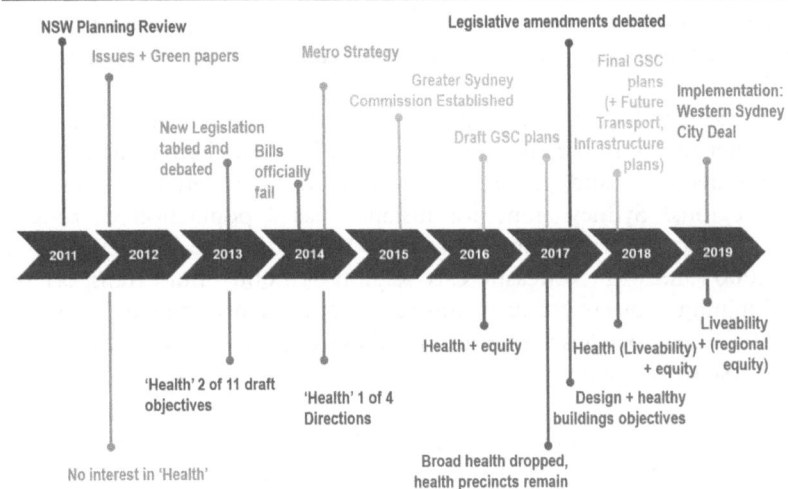

Fig. 6.1 Changes to NSW Urban and Regional Policy over the life of this research

explicit opportunity for influencing the delivery of the strategic intent of the planning system. The reality is much murkier, I go on to show. But 'development assessment' captures any type of 'development' from a single dwelling (house) to massive infrastructure projects. I was less interested in the former largely because my primary interest is the health of whole populations, not individual dwellings (although yes, I hear you, these can be aggregated up at a population level). I have also had a long-standing interest in health impact assessment, and with that came an interest in environmental impact assessment (Harris et al., 2015). For this research, my focus was a category of very large infrastructure projects that underwent a type of development assessment termed 'Environmental Assessments' (same process as an environmental impact assessment). The projects covered under this process are defined under the legislation as 'major', 'state significant developments' or 'state significant', 'or critical state' infrastructure. The triggers for such developments were usually their geographic and financial size. Put simply, they mattered for the economic development of the state. Given that there were a great many types of major development occurring at any one time, I decided to focus my attention on what was important politically at that time. This political angle led me to focus on urban transport infrastructure projects as one form of development, and, to add a regional flavour, coal mining projects as the other.

The size and scale of these initiatives ought to be recognised up front. My interest, as stated, is population health. What better than investigating decisions and processes that will go on to affect whole cities and regions? Sydney alone for instance has a population of roughly 5.5 million. Western Sydney is around 1 million. The Hunter Valley is 270,000 (and with Newcastle City Region 600,000). Both transport and coal mining projects produce emissions that influence the whole planet.

The **research questions** followed these outlined aspects of the planning system, as follows:

- What organisational and procedural processes led to effective cross-sectoral action for health within the NSW land-use planning system following health being recognised as important in the 2011–13 review of the planning legislation?
- Following the 2011–2013 review, how, why and to what extent were health-related issues, including health equity, taken up and operationalised in two core components of the land-use planning system: strategic level 'plan-making' and 'development assessment' of major development projects?

Specific objectives of the research program were to:

- Inform health policy and practice in Australia and internationally by providing evidence of the requirements to influence health being included in the strategic legislative and policy and planning business of a non-health sector.
- Identify the roles and requirements within the health system to engage effectively with land-use planning to develop healthy built environments.
- Develop and test a framework for understanding effective cross-sectoral action for health within complex and dynamic policy systems.

- Develop and test an analytical framework for evaluating land-use plans for their health impact.

The majority of the research focussed on NSW. However, just as I received my own funding for the above research, I also became part of two other successfully funded research enterprises. That additional focus allowed me to compare other jurisdictions, particularly Adelaide, South Australia (around 1.3 million people).

ANALYTIC FRAMEWORK

I have detailed the methodology and analytic frameworks in the first part of this book. Here, I recap briefly with the focus on the NSW planning system.

Realist methodology investigates and explains complex problems by developing propositions about 'conditions' and 'mechanisms' which lead to 'outcomes' or 'events' (Pawson & Tilley, 1997; Sayer, 2000). To do this, realist analysis begins by breaking down the problem under investigation into its essential parts (Sayer, 1992). As introduced already, essentially the NSW land-use system has two functions which this research will focus on: 'plan-making', where regional, sub-regional and local plans are developed; and 'development assessment' which is the regulated process of assessing and considering for approval an application for a development project.

Additionally—as shown in part I of this book—policy development is rarely linear or rational but has three core units of analysis (presented in Fig. 5.1 Chapter 5): *ideas, actors and structures,* with additional elements of *processes, decisions and choices, outcomes and event, governance and power,* and *time.* These units of analysis formed the basis of explanations about the 'conditions' and 'mechanisms' which led to the outcome of health being included (and how and to what extent) across the essential aspects of the land-use planning system.

PROGRAM OF WORK AND METHODS

The research program incorporated overlapping stages of work following case-study design (Yin, 2012).

I built the program around a series of case studies that represented the various core dynamics of a land-use planning system. A case study is an in-depth study of a single unit, or a group of units, where the researcher's aim is to elucidate features of a larger class of similar phenomena (Yin, 2012). Case-study designs are recognised in public health social science research as providing important insight where other designs (e.g. controlled trials) are not possible (Petticrew et al., 2009). Multiple explanatory case studies focus on how and why phenomena occur, where each case demonstrates or uncovers specific findings which are then either demonstrated or not in other cases.

Data collection included publicly available documentation, including associated media coverage (print and social), and qualitative data collection via purposively sampled interviews with from five to ten participants per case and focus groups where useful and possible ($n = 92$) people.

Data analysis was conducted using NVIVO software (QSR International Pty Ltd.). Content analysis allowed a focus on how 'health' was included and conceptualised in documents (e.g. as 'health' or 'wellbeing' or 'environmental health' or 'health protection' or 'health promotion' or 'sustainability and health' or 'disadvantage'). Interview data was analysed using a variety of qualitative approaches to develop explanations and propositions about conditions and mechanisms which led to outcomes and events.

This empirical analysis was substantially integrated with critical theory from a range of disciplines including political science, public administration, planning and urban studies.

The research proceeded over stages, as follows.

Stage one *(2015)*: **How, why and to what extent did health became an objective in the 2011–2013 NSW review of land-use planning legislation?**
Stage two *(2015–2017)*: **The extent to which health and health equity concerns are considered in plan-making between 2015 and 2017, and what factors impeded or encouraged this happening.**
Stage three *(2015–2018)*: **How, why and the extent to which health is included in environmental assessments and approval processes for Major Projects in NSW?**

I added the Western Sydney City Deal to this aspect of the work, although this was funded through a National Health and Medical Research Council Centre for Research Excellence (Policy Research on the Social Determinant of Health Equity) that I was part of.

Stage four: Infrastructure policy in Australia *(2016–2017).*
An additional stage added during the research focussed on infrastructure policymaking. Our documentary analysis in stage one and interviews in stage three suggested that infrastructure should become an core object of the research. With additional funding from Sydney University, we went about analysing infrastructure plans and conducting interviews with leading infrastructure policy makers across the country.

Stage five: Urban planning policies across Australia/Comparing Master Plans in Sydney and Adelaide (2016–2017).
Additional related research with colleagues at Flinders University in South Australia was funded as an Australian Research Council Discovery project. My work had two phases. First was an analysis of 108 current (between March 2016 and February 2017) policies and legislation from state, territory and federal governments collected from departmental websites. The documents were analysed thematically to ascertain whether and how they addressed the social determinants of health and health equity. We then compared the 2012 New South Wales Long Term Transport Master Plan and the (2017) Thirty Year Plan for Greater Adelaide in South Australia (SA). We mixed findings from the documentary analysis with 21 interviews (10 in NSW and 11 in SA).

CASE-STUDY DESIGN—MULTIPLE EXPLANATORY CASE STUDIES

Yin (2012) differentiates between single cases, multiple cases, descriptive, exploratory and explanatory analysis. As shown in Chapter 4, explanation focussing on 'how and why' is preferred in critical realism over description of 'what?'. I therefore focussed on explanatory case-study design using multiple cases. Each case demonstrated or uncovered specific findings which were then replicated, or not, in further cases. In terms of conditions, the aim was to explain the case and the context(s) surrounding the case(s). Within each case were comparable units of analysis—the elements of the policy cube presented in Chapter 5.

DATA COLLECTION

The research used tools and methods that are standard for in-depth field-work of real world, complex, policymaking (Cairney et al., 2019). Two methods, documentary analysis and stakeholder interviews, were core to the program (see Table 6.1 at the end of the chapter). *Document analysis* has long been recognised a crucial method for policy analysis research (Sabatier, 1988). *In-depth stakeholder interviews* are also a standard policy analysis method (Kingdon, 2011).

DOCUMENTARY ANALYSIS

We[1] undertook documentary analysis for each stage of the program. Policy documents are incredibly useful and insightful windows on the world of policymaking. They are also often publicly available. Documents present the core ideas that policy makers want the public to see, but at the same time serve to present the values and interests that produce those ideas, and the structured rules and mandates that allow those ideas to be presented. Indeed, what we tended to do was to undertake and publish the documentary analysis first, followed by a deeper investigation using interviews and theory. Most stages focussed on a mix of content and thematic analysis. We also included discourse analysis in the strategic planning phases, one of which (WSCD) was a critical discourse analysis (Fairclough, 2003) that explicitly analysed the policy document against existing theoretical frameworks.

Overall, we analysed around 250 documents ranging in length from a few pages to 1000s. The lightest touch was applied in the infrastructure phase when we merely searched for the use of the word 'health' in three State level infrastructure plans. At the other end of the scale were environmental impact statements and the documents produced from an environmental assessment. These reports are often 1000s of pages and are not for the fainthearted. In some stages, we included Hansard recordings of parliamentary proceedings and government documents accessed through open access to information processes (including emails, internal reports and minutes of meetings).

---

[1] Please note that from this point in the book, I begin to use the term 'we' rather than 'I'. I did not collect and analyse data alone! 'I' is retained in instances where I led the data collection and analysis.

The analytic frameworks were slightly different for each phase or project—and can be seen in the source papers we wrote (Baum, Delany-Crowe et al., 2018; Harris et al., 2016; Hresc et al., 2018, Riley, Sainsbury et al., 2019; Riley et al., 2017).

INTERVIEWS

Interview participants were almost always sampled purposively (Rubin & Rubin, 2011). The main inclusion criteria were being an influential or major stakeholder in the specific case or topic of investigation. We also used snowball sampling from the original informants.

Of 114 invited, 92 took part (81% response rate). Of those who did not take part around 1/3 did not respond to requests, and 2/3 indicated they were not sufficiently involved in the case to take part (sometimes then suggesting another person). I am taking a liberty by not detailing participants here. Those details can be found in the original academic papers produced at each point in the research. I personally conducted all the NSW interviews bar a couple on the 2012 Transport Masterplan. Nearly all were face to face.

Interviews were designed as conversations (from 15 to 90 min). The interviews were essentially designed around the three core a priori institutionalist factors: structures (rules and mandates governing practice), actors (stakeholders and networks) and ideas (the content of policy). Conversations are crucial. Being relaxed about the format of the interview elicits better data than a formal question by question approach. The point is to get the informant to open up. Participants were usually provided a draft interview schedule prior to the meeting (for ethical approval reasons plus to get them to think through the complexities). My experience is that people are more than willing to chat about the complexities of their work. However, silences need attending to. Prompts for conditions and mechanisms as well as questions that take a critical angle are also challenges to watch out for.

The realist methodologist Ray Pawson introduces the core elements to the realist interview I ascribe to (Pawson, 1996; Pawson & Tilley, 1997). I've often found that informants will talk through most of the questions in an interview schedule even if the conversation unfolds in an unstructured manner. If they don't then questions not yet responded to can be returned to before the interview is up. Finally, my experience with interviews is that each interview is a game of trying to get information the

Table 6.1 Overview of research program

Focus area	Background	RQ	Case(s)	Detail	'Health' finding	Documents included	Interviews (n = 92)	Pub(s)
Legislative advocacy	The health advocacy work that occurred to influence the 2011–2013 legislative reforms of the NSW planning system was, at that time, a world first for healthy public policy. It is impossible to underestimate the advocacy challenge of influencing legislation in place for nearly 50 years without any reference to human health	How and why did health come to be incorporated in the 2011–2013 review of the NSW planning system? What lessons can be learnt from this case about high level, strategic, legislative advocacy for health?	2011–2013 review of the NSW planning system	Investigated advocacy that led to the inclusion of health in the Bill tabled to Parliament in 2013 and the wider reform process	Health had moment in the sun but ultimately not included explicitly in legislation	Random samples of public submissions to the review (total = 7000 over 3 phases): -31 from 19 different health focused agencies -24 from 7 different 'key stakeholder' agencies -47 from 47 other agencies Hansard recordings of parliamentary proceedings Government documents accessed through open access to information processes (including email, internal reports and minutes of meetings)	9 interviews and a focus group	Harris et al. (2016), Harris, Kent et al. (2018a, 2018b), Kent, Harris et al. (2018a, 2018b)
Strategic Planning 1	Australian urban or metropolitan strategic spatial planning has evolved to be a core public policy activity through which state governments (the middle layer of Australia's federated government system). Health is historically not a focus beyond hospital infrastructure	How and why health was positioned in strategic land-use planning in Sydney during this 2014–2018 period?	Sydney City (region) plans Sydney District level plans	Two instances of strategic spatial planning in Sydney across the four-year study period allowed us to investigate how health was considered, and why, over time and if there were any differences	'Health' considered but not with no actions or mechanism to make real. Preference for hospital precincts	2 × regional plans 5 × district plans	11 interviews	Harris, Kent et al. (2020a, 2020b)

Focus area	Background	RQ	Case(s)	Detail	'Health' finding	Documents included	Interviews (n = 92)	Pub(s)
Strategic Planning 2	Strategic spatial plans attempt to coordinate the medium- to long-term development of city regions that include inner cities, suburbs and peri-urban surrounds. They typically include one or more overarching macro-level normative social, environmental and/or economic goals as well as objectives that advance them	What are the connections between the two plans and aspects of liveability that have direct benefits for social determinants of health?	NSW transport masterplan (2012) Greater Adelaide (2017)	How health and social determinants are considered and why	Some health focus especially Adelaide. Liveability the entry point for health but requires equity focus	Two plans	21 Interviews	McGreevy et al. (2019), McGreevy, Harris et al. (2020a, 2020b) McGreevy, Harris et al. (2020a, 2020b)
Environmental Assessments 1: Transport mega-projects in Sydney and Adelaide	The transport and health impact evidence base is descriptive and has developed largely in the absence of a deep understanding of the of the decisions that inform major transport decisions. Environmental impact assessment (EIA) is one of these procedures. In Australia, the EIA process is called Environmental Assessment (EA)	'How, why, and to what extent, is human health considered in environmental assessments of major transport infrastructure projects?' 'What were the main influences behind how health was included?'	NSW: NorthConnex, CBD and South East Light Rail (CSELR), WestConnex M4 East South Australia: 2010 Darlington Upgrade	Technical inclusion of health impacts in EAs for transport, and the institutional dynamics of how and why health was included or not	Health risks the focus rather than broad range of health impacts	Environmental Impact Statements or equivalent for each case, requirements or guidance issued, reports based on community submissions, and broader approvals documentation	15 Interviews (Sydney projects only)	Harris, Riley et al. (2018a, 2018b) and Riley et al.(2017)

(continued)

Table 6.1 (continued)

Focus area	Background	RQ	Case(s)	Detail	'Health' finding	Documents included	Interviews (n = 92)	Pub(s)
Environmental Assessments 2: Coal mining in NSW	Unclear how effectively coal mining EAs assess health and wellbeing issues and whether the focus is too narrow to address the social determinants of health (SDH) and health equity as a means of attaining the health promotion focus	How and to what extent are health, wellbeing and equity issues considered in environmental impact assessments (EIAs) of major coal mining projects in New South Wales, Australia. What influences the inclusion of health issues in environmental assessments of coal mining projects in NSW, Australia?	Coal mining in New South Wales	Technical inclusion of health impacts in EAs for coal mining, and the institutional dynamics of how and why health was included or not	Health risks the focus rather than broad range of health impacts	Environmental impact statements, media articles Specific EAs for documentary analysis were: Watermark Coal Project—opencut mine. Warkworth Continuation—opencut mine. Mandalong Southern Extension—underground mine	15 interviews	Hresc et al. (2018) Riley, Sainsbury et al. (2019), Harris et al. and (2021)
Infrastructure	'Infrastructure' is a global 'multi-trillion dollar market' that presents many opportunities to improve public health and sustainable development Infrastructure policymaking has yet to be investigated as a policy sector from a healthy public policy perspective	What infrastructure policy is, what assumptions lie behind it, what the influences are on the way it functions, and what its actual and potential connections to and tensions with public health might be?	Australian infrastructure policy and planning	Institutional approach to investigate how infrastructure and health and wellbeing, as part of the sustainable development goals, are conceptualised in Australian infrastructure policy and planning	Health not understood or considered	Australian Infrastructure Plan (2016) Victoria's draft 30-year infrastructure strategy (2016) NSW State Infrastructure Strategy Update (2014)	10 interviews with senior practising infrastructure policy makers and experts across Australia	Harris, Riley et al. (2020a, 2020b)
Regional plan implementation	'City Deals' are new governance instruments for urban development. Despite a vast evidence base urban and regional factors with health equity, little research applies a health equity lens to urban policymaking	To what extent, and why, did the implementation planning of the Western Sydney City Deal consider health equity?'	Western Sydney City Deal	Whether or not the implementation of the Western Sydney City Deal allowed for consideration of health equity. Emphasis on goals and objectives, governance, and place-making	Health considered as part of liveability. Equity not considered	2018 implementation plan, subsequent annual reporting, publicly available information, media articles	12 interviews	Friel, Townsend et al. (2021) and Harris, Fisher et al. (2022)

respondent is either willing to give this up or not—see also (Smith, 2006). Also, at the end of the day, interviews are empirical; more work is always required to go deeper than what an informant or set of interview data can or will reveal.

SUMMARY

This chapter has provided the protocol for the research reported over the rest of this section of the book. As with any type of case-study inquiry, presenting a protocol does not only introduce methodology and methods. It also provides a centrepiece from which to begin to consider the internal validity of the findings in the rest of the research. By writing in some of the details involved in data collection and then data analysis, I supported claims to validity by identifying the core dynamics of the research process. The book now turns to the analytic resolution section of the research where the focus is unpacking the empirical dimensions of the phenomenon under investigation (Table 6.1).

REFERENCES

Baum, F., Delany-Crowe, T., Fisher, M., MacDougall, C., Harris, P. McDermott, D.,& Marinova, D. (2018). Qualitative protocol for understanding the contribution of Australian policy in the urban planning, justice, energy and environment sectors to promoting health and health equity. *BMJ Open 8*(9).

Cairney, P., Heikkila, T., & Wood, M. (2019). *Making policy in a complex world.* Cambridge University Press.

Dodson, J. (2017). The global infrastructure turn and urban practice. *Urban Policy and Research, 35*(1), 87–92.

Fairclough, N. (2003). *Analysing discourse: Textual analysis for social research.* Psychology Press.

Friel, S., Townsend, B., Fisher, M., Harris, P., Freeman, T., Baum, F. J. (2021). Power and the people's health. *Social Science and Medicine, 282*(August), 114173.

Harris, P., Viliani, F., & Spickett, J. (2015). Assessing health impacts within environmental impact assessments: An opportunity for public health globally which must not remain missed. *International Journal of Environmental Research and Public Health, 12*(1), 1044–1049.

Harris, P., Kent, J., Sainsbury, P., Marie-Thow, A., Baum, F., Friel, S., & McCue, P. (2018a). Creating 'healthy built environment' legislation in Australia; A policy analysis. *Health Promotion International, 33*(6), 1090–1100.

Harris, P., Riley, E., Sainsbury, P., Kent, J., & Baum, F. (2018b). Including health in environmental impact assessments of three mega transport projects in Sydney, Australia: A critical, institutional, analysis. *Environmental Impact Assessment Review 68*(Supplement C): 109–116.

Harris, P., Kent, J., Sainsbury, P., Riley, E., Sharma, N., & Harris, E. (2020a). Healthy urban planning: an institutional policy analysis of strategic planning in Sydney, Australia. *Health Promotion International 35*(5).

Harris, P., Riley, E., Dawson, A., Friel, S., & Lawson, K. (2020b). "Stop talking around projects and talk about solutions": Positioning health within infrastructure policy to achieve the Sustainable Development Goals. *Health Policy, 124*(6), 591–598.

Harris, P., Kent, J., Sainsbury, P., & Thow, A.-M. (2016). Framing health for land-use planning legislation: A qualitative descriptive content analysis. *Social Science & Medicine, 148*, 42–51.

Harris, P., McManus, P., Sainsbury, P., Viliani, F., & Riley, E. (2021). The institutional dynamics behind limited human health considerations in environmental assessments of coal mining projects in New South Wales, Australia. *Environmental Impact Assessment Review, 86*, 106473.

Harris, P. J., Harris-Roxas, B. F., & Harris, E. (2007). An overview of the regulatory planning system in New South Wales: Identifying points of intervention for health impact assessment and consideration of health impacts. *New South Wales Public Health Bulletin, 18*(10), 188–191.

Hresc, J., Riley, E., & Harris, P. (2018). Mining project's economic impact on local communities, as a social determinant of health: A documentary analysis of environmental impact statements. *Environmental Impact Assessment Review, 72*, 64–70.

Kent, J. L., Harris, P., Sainsbury, P., Baum, F., McCue, P., & Thompson, S. (2018). Influencing urban planning policy: An exploration from the perspective of public health. *Urban Policy and Research, 36*(1), 20–34.

Kingdon, J. W. (2011). *Agendas, alternatives, and public policies* (3rd ed.). Ill, Pearson Education Inc.

McGreevy, M., Harris, P., Delaney-Crowe, T., Fisher, M., Sainsbury, P., & Baum, F. (2020a). The power of collaborative planning: How a health and planning collaboration facilitated integration of health goals in the 30-year plan for Greater Adelaide. *Urban Policy and Research, 38* (3), 262–275.

McGreevy, M., Harris, P., Delaney-Crowe, T., Fisher, M., Sainsbury, P., Riley, E., & Baum, F. (2020b). How well do Australian government urban planning policies respond to the social determinants of health and health equity? *J Land Use Policy, 99*, 105053.

McGreevy, M., Harris, P., Delany-Crowe, T., Fisher, M., Sainsbury, P., & Baum, F. (2019). Can health and health equity be advanced by urban planning strategies designed to advance global competitiveness? Lessons from two Australian case studies. *Social Science & Medicine, 242,* 112594.

NSW Government Office of the Government Architect. (2018). *Better Placed,* from https://www.governmentarchitect.nsw.gov.au/policies/better-placed.

Pawson, R. (1996). Theorizing the interview. *British Journal of Sociology:* 295–314.

Pawson, R., & Tilley, N. (1997). *Realistic evaluation.* Sage.

Petticrew, M., Tugwell, P., Welch, V., Ueffing, E., Kristjansson, E., Armstrong, R., Doyle, J., & Waters, E. (2009). Better evidence about wicked issues in tackling health inequities. *Journal of Public Health, 31*(3), 453–456.

Riley, E., Harris, P., Kent, J., Sainsbury, P., Lane, A., & Baum, F. (2017). Including health in environmental assessments of major transport infrastructure projects: A documentary analysis. *International Journal of Health Policy and Management, 7*(2), 144–153.

Riley, E., Sainsbury, P., McManus, P., Colagiuri, R., Viliani, F., Dawson, A., Duncan, E., Stone, Y., Pham, T., & Harris, P. (2019). Including health impacts in environmental impact assessments for three Australian coal-mining projects: a documentary analysis. *Health Promotion International, 35*(3), 449–457.

Rubin, H. J., & Rubin, I. S. (2011). *Qualitative interviewing: The art of hearing data.* Sage.

Sabatier, P. A. (1988). An advocacy coalition framework of policy change and the role of policy-oriented learning therein. *Policy Sciences, 21*(2), 129–168.

Sayer, A. (1992). *Method in social science: A realist approach* (2nd ed.). Routledge.

Sayer, A. (2000). *Realism and social science,* Sage.

Smith, K. E. (2006). Problematising power relations in 'elite' interviews. *Geoforum, 37*(4), 643–653.

Yin, R. K. (2012). *Case study research: Design and methods.* Sage.

CHAPTER 7

Empirical Data

This chapter covers research steps one and two, previously introduced in Chapter 4. I present empirically focussed data analysis across the case studies (see Table 6.1 Chapter 6). I do this against the core constructs introduced in Chapter 5: Actors, Structures, Ideas and Processes.

By the time I drafted this book I had produced a series of stand-alone articles, to which I refer throughout. Writing the book became a whole new task in synthesising the program's findings. To write up this chapter, for instance, I went back to the coding undertaken in NVIVO (QSR International Pty Ltd.) across the research program. I focussed on relations and patterns rather than numerical rates (see Sayer, 1992, 2000). I first, however, used the numbers of codes to alert me to when an issue or code was raised more often both within a case and across the five cases. I then qualitatively checked whether that issue connected with other similar codes that may have had fewer instance of coding. I then went back into the data itself to see how that issue was expressed, sometimes checking if the coding was right or needed changing to reflect the data. This allowed me to come up with the themes (each theme is in **bold**) presented below.

The main outcome measure was how health was included (or not) in the various cases and levels of policymaking. The task was to disassemble the data against the core institutional constructs, and in doing so describe

P. Harris, *Illuminating Policy for Health*, Palgrave Studies
in Public Health Policy Research,
https://doi.org/10.1007/978-3-031-13199-8_7

the policy system under scrutiny. For the jobbing researcher under pressure to publish or perish, this surface level empirical analysis, done well and systematically, can be published on its own; indeed much research published today happens at similar surface levels.

ACTORS

Greater Sydney Commission. The Greater Sydney Commission (GSC) ended up a major focus of the research. In many ways, Commissions are Policy Instruments (Howlett et al., 2009) set up to provide independent advice or work through complex problems. The GSC was given the task of setting up integrated planning across traditional siloed ways of working, and crucially to link that planning to the delivery of infrastructure. As such, the GSC was the central player in the analysis of strategic planning (with the exception of the transport strategy), although was not involved in the Environmental Assessment cases as this was not part of their remit.

The community was a cross cutting actor. Community was discussed mainly in terms of the challenges with effective engagement in planning and environmental Assessment. From a health perspective, this was perhaps the pre-eminent issue in the case studies that leant closer to implementation: Environmental Assessment and Western Sydney City Deal. An interesting counter point was the crucial role that the public played in the legislative case study, although the advocates did not use the health argument as part of their strategy (see ideas). In general, community input was often piecemeal and dismissed as biased by those who were required to engage with them. Communities in turn distrusted institutionalised processes as biased against them.

The government was identified as a crucial actor. All the cases involved particular government agencies as having influential roles, particularly the Department of Planning and to a lesser extent the Department/Ministry of Health. The Department of Transport and the Roads and Maritime services had a particular role in one of the strategic planning cases, and also acted as an influential powerful actor across all the cases. Transport held more power, and a bigger budget, than Planning. Budgeting roads or even particular transport infrastructure projects over and above strategic planning or the local infrastructure network became a major structural problem from a population health perspective. Within government, Treasury and Cabinet held ultimate power. The interests of both set the ideas in motion that flow through the system to processes and then decisions that were made and funded. Those interests also influenced the parameters of the technical procedures—business cases, EAs—that the system used to fulfil these tasks. Needless to say, both Treasury and Cabinet essentially took a financial cost lens. From a health perspective, that lens zeroed in on health as hospital infrastructure. Health infrastructure, for instance, was described as a powerful player from the health sector (see next) but was expected to engage in urban and regional planning with a remit focussed on hospitals.

The Federated Australian government system was also described as playing a profound, albeit often invisible, influence on urban policy. The **Federal government** had a major role as a funder of very large infrastructure projects, as well as a role in trying to shift policy and practice towards better competencies through improved guidance and so forth. The traditional lack of policy interest in urban policy by the Federal government hung heavily over all the data analysis. So too their active interest in transport and other (minus the urban) 'economic' infrastructure types. Notably, the interest of the Federal government in the airport in Western Sydney became the crucial opportunity for better linking infrastructure and the development of Western Sydney.

Finally, from a government perspective, **local government** was coded across all the cases. **Local councils** in NSW were removed in the 2000s from being formally involved in the statutory process for assessing very large state significant infrastructure. At best, councils lobbied or made submissions but were mostly sidelined from major decisions. Local councils were however discussed a crucial point of engagement for the district planning that underpinned the work of the GSC. Councils were also driving forces behind the Western Sydney City Deal and thus integral to that case analysis. However, because of the context in NSW and our focus on strategic plans and state significant projects, both of which crossed local council boundaries, the internal machinations of specific local governments were less of a focus.

The **health sector**, unsurprisingly, was identified as an organisational level actor. The influence of the health sector on the inclusion of health waxed and waned. For instance, several 'wins' for health happened without health sector leadership. Health advocates, mostly led by those working outside the formal health sector, were the fundamental catalyst for initially including health in the failed 2011–2013 draft legislative reform (Harris, Kent et al., 2018). Health sector engagement did help position health in the strategic plans although this input ultimately tended towards hospital infrastructure (Harris, Kent et al., 2020a, 2020b, 2020c). Health was included as the primary goal of a major 'place based' policy, but no specific health sector stakeholders were listed in that document as being involved (NSW Government Office of the Government Architect, 2018). Health sector engagement in environmental Assessments almost exclusively focussed on environmental risks, with questionable influence on fundamental project decisions (Harris, McManus et al., 2021; Harris, Riley et al., 2018a, 2018b, Hresc et al., 2018, Riley, Sainsbury et al., 2019; Riley et al., 2017). However, an active and interested health sector did make a difference. For instance, EAs default to health risk assessment directly as a result of health department interests. In an different example, when comparing NSW and South Australia, the South Australian 'health in all policies unit' impacted on the content of the SA plan in more overt ways than the more diffuse health input in the NSW transport plan (McGreevy et al., 2019, McGreevy, Harris et al., 2020a, 2020b, 2020c).

Concerning **individuals**, specific Ministers and their staffers were influential. This influence did not tend to focus on health, but rather set up the opportunities and mechanisms for health or health-related issues to be included or excluded. The Planning Minister was crucial. A particular Minister, Rob Stokes, became particularly influential during the life of the research. A Planner by professional background, Minister Stokes opened up institutional opportunities for health input; some eventuating, some not. He oversaw the Greater Sydney Commission to re-work strategic Sydney plans and deliver legislative requirements to implement strategic/spatial land use planning by connecting this with infrastructure plans and funding. He also oversaw setting up the concept of design-led, place-based planning that could be a catalyst for health-focussed planning. However, the relative lack of power of the Planning portfolio comparted to other Ministries was notable. A good relationship for any Minister with the Premier was fundamental: ultimate power belongs to the Premier as the elected head of state government.

A raft of **particular individuals** played powerful roles in opening up or shifting the system to be more or less open to health input. These individuals worked within and outside of government. They had greater or lesser influence depending on the case at hand. Participants often identified the tension between bureaucrats and ministerial offices or politician's staffers. These tensions manifested in the regular back and forth about particular

ideas and interests that were inserted by bureaucrats only to be deleted by ministerial offices, then reinserted and so on and so forth.

A core finding how groups of particular individuals set urban planning and infrastructure agendas. This work included garnering the support of the Premier and relevant ministers—or occurred within close circles to the government and its agenda. For example, we tracked the idea of Australia's largest infrastructure (>$22 Billion) project, the WestConnex road/tunnel, to a (35 page) document produced by Infrastructure NSW in 2012.[1] This almost inconspicuous document supports an observation of the power of individuals by one (anonymous) participant:

> *Interviewer* And then WestConnex comes along. How did that interact with what was going on in terms of the master plan?
> *Participant*: It didn't. No. Because what [then Premier] 'POLITICIAN X'[2] had said was 'whichever one road project Infrastructure NSW selects I will build'. That was his political campaign promise. And he had in mind two competing projects....So, he thought it was one [motorway] or the other [motorway]. But of course 'POLITICIAN Y' [former Premier], who just happened to be on the board of Infrastructure NSW with 'BUSINESS LEADER' [the head of a construction firm] said to him, 'If we draw this line between the two it's only one road, isn't it?' And everybody went, 'Hmm, good idea'. That was the extent of their planning for WestConnex.

In a nutshell, this comment and the supporting documents suggest a particularly powerful group of individuals in and outside of government cemented the idea of Australia's largest infrastructure investment as a policy reality with next to no process, transparency, accountability or scrutiny. The power of several individuals—outside of any formal planning process for the city—created an infrastructure juggernaut that will transform a city for over 100 years with profound implications for health and wellbeing. ALL subsequent processes and decisions associated with WestConnex occurred within the parameters of that fundamental decision for a single, massive, costly, road (Haughton & McManus, 2019; McManus & Haughton, 2021; Robertson et al., 2021; Searle & Legacy,

---

[1] http://www.infrastructure.nsw.gov.au/media/1160/insw_tfnsw_and_roads_and_mar itime_services_wcx_25_sept_2012_final_120927.pdf (Accessed 14 July 20).

[2] Names removed.

2021). For instance, the 2014 report by the Audit Office of NSW[3] found failure to comply with the Major Projects Assurance Framework and that the governance arrangements failed to clearly separate those responsible for delivery, commissioning and assurance. The report states:

> Reliance was placed on steering committees and boards with responsibility for project delivery to also provide independent assurance to the Government. There is a fundamental conflict in such an arrangement. A steering committee or board with delivery responsibility cannot provide truly independent advice to government.

Ideas overlap with actors, of course. The need for transport infrastructure investment in Sydney, on the back of decades of policy inaction, was identified by most participants. The essential problem was whether a $22 Billion road was a better investment than investing in the public transport network across the city, especially in the West where public transport infrastructure was and remains notoriously bad. This is crucial from a health perspective where the evidence suggests roads create poor health outcomes, and that instead of more roads a mix of transport options is required to improve health impacts (Litman, 2013). The original report notably argues that 'WestConnex must be more than a road' (p. 9). There is no evidence from my or other research that this commitment has eventuated.

The **role of industry** was crucial. Development does not happen without industry. The health agenda in some instances is pro-industry—liveability for instance can help developers as well as impact positively on the public (Hooper, Foster et al., 2020). But health focussed planning is not always industry enabling. For instance, a health framing often questions the impact of large infrastructure projects on local communities. Overall, balancing private with public actor engagement emerged as a tension that lies at the heart of healthy urban planning.

Others was a category I used to cover the range of other stakeholders involved. These people included consultants (for technical tasks in particular like EAs), invited experts and/or commissioned experts, non-government organisations, as well as other sectors or service providers—for instance, the social services sector. **Consultancy firms** emerged as

---

[3] https://www.audit.nsw.gov.au/our-work/reports/performance-audit-insights-key-findings-from-2014-2018 Accessed 14/07/20.

extremely powerful actors. Consultancy firms were clearly used by government as the primary point for knowledge creation or affirmation (more on affirmation later).

Finally, overlapping with governance, **networks and coalitions** also emerged clearly as a theme from the data. Essentially, the data suggest there is power in groups that works largely off the back of individual leadership and effort. There was the sense that groups form either naturally or strategically (or formally as committees or advisory groups) around various issues. Health was not often front and centre of these groups, but their actions and interests led to the opportunities for a health agenda or health input to exploit. 'Health' had a creeping, incremental (see ideas), relevance to these groups, particularly through the concept of liveability.

STRUCTURES

Rules and mandates were coded as a fundamental structural influence. This is unsurprising, recalling that institutional theory defines institutional structures essentially as rules and mandates that flow through systems (Cairney et al., 2019; Peters, 2019). Of note here is that 'ideas' (see next) were coded often as exerting influences throughout the system as rules and mandates.

At a meta level, for instance, the research occurred at a time when **a shift to a 'whole of government approach to city making'** (participant, strategic planning project) was becoming a reality. In the past, the much vaunted idea of **integrated planning** (planning meets infrastructure delivery by engaging different agencies) was repeatedly and historically hobbled by the siloed and power laden institutional set up of government. Planning was a relatively powerless portfolio when compared with Transport, for instance. Thus in 2013 at the start of the research integrated planning was a pipe dream. But by the end the Sydney region (and by extension the district plans which fed off this) had been produced 'concurrently' with the State transport strategy and the State Infrastructure strategy. That shift to integrated planning represented a golden window of opportunity for health advocates. Integrated planning, as already noted, has been positioned as institutional requirement to improve health and wellbeing in cities (Giles-Corti et al., 2016). During the decade covered in this research, an institutionalised connection to health ideas, collaborations and outcomes never really eventuated. Understanding why is, of course, the topic of the rest of the book.

The novel mandate of integrated planning practice as an opportunity to position health in the system butted up against **'a history of previous institutional decisions'**. Across the cases, participants identified a historical tendency across senior or high levels of government to see health as unimportant. A good example of this is that 'health' was historically viewed within the Department of Planning as 'too theoretical', meaning it was not practical or pragmatic enough to action as a policy mandate. That lack of support trickled down through the system. The emphasis at a strategic/spatial infrastructure level tended to remain on hospital infrastructure precincts rather than a healthy city or even healthy environment to keep people out of hospital. And at the project level there was no discernible shift in practice, despite guidance being issued that included conducting health impact assessments for critical state infrastructure, to consider the range of health impacts that inevitably come with such mega-projects.

This history of institutional decisions was structurally compounded by the ongoing problem of **silos** within government agencies. Several participants across the research expressed frustration that the much vaunted ideal of 'creating great places'—place-making—was continually undermined by an inability to or interest in share budgets across agencies or levels of government. One participant observed how much of the work attempting to shift the planning system towards a more progressive urban model—integrated planning, governance and so forth—was in fact window dressing, and that **real structural change had yet to occur** at a macro level.

The elemental structural driver for the planning system was described under the theme of **economic drivers**. At its most stark, this was described as.

'Free market thinking with minimal government interference' (participant, strategic planning).

The role of **the market** was a dominant force both within and external government (see governance next). At the highest levels, the dominant mandate behind the planning system was clearly oriented towards market led economic growth to managing population growth, creating jobs and providing housing. Transport, for example, was described in purely economic[4] terms:

> *Our economy has changed, our economy is not a manufacturing economy, it's a knowledge economy, it's very much dependent on the CBDs, CBDs are very much dependent on workers being able to access them. That is dependent on public transport by and large and so we're seeing in Sydney, Melbourne and Brisbane now moves towards substantial step change in the public transport networks. Big investments in metro rail which is where we need to go for our cities to be competitive.*

(Participant, infra)

There was a view that land use, or the built environment, was open to market mechanisms such that infrastructure began to 'fund itself' (Participant infra). This ability for a market 'platform' behind infrastructure, as it was described, varied from sector to sector. Land transport infrastructure was explained as currently largely dependent on government because market-based reform had yet to happen in that sector. Energy, in contrast, was largely private sector funded based on a market model for delivery, but as a sector is ultimately governed by government policy and regulation.

Figures 7.1 and 7.2 show some of the politicisation and community backlash towards the market led infrastructure agenda.

As a structural mandate, providing **infrastructure** was explained as political shorthand for 'getting the state moving' (participant, strategic planning) and a fundamental facilitator of society (Harris, Riley et al., 2020a, 2020b, 2020c). However, the tension became clear between delivering infrastructure as an economic 'asset' and its role in providing a 'service'. This tension in turn opens a pandora's box of issues from a public health perspective.

Central to this already heady structural mix is **governance**. I cannot describe governance sufficiently without theory. Empirically, urban governance tended to be explained as what the role of government vis-a-vis the private sector was. The community, notably, tended not to feature as prominently. Government tended to be seen as representing communities

---

[4] *Theory really helps at this point. I am however, purposefully holding back. Doing so might be frustrating for some readers, but this clear need for theory supports the type of analysis advocated for in the book. You can of course jump ahead.*

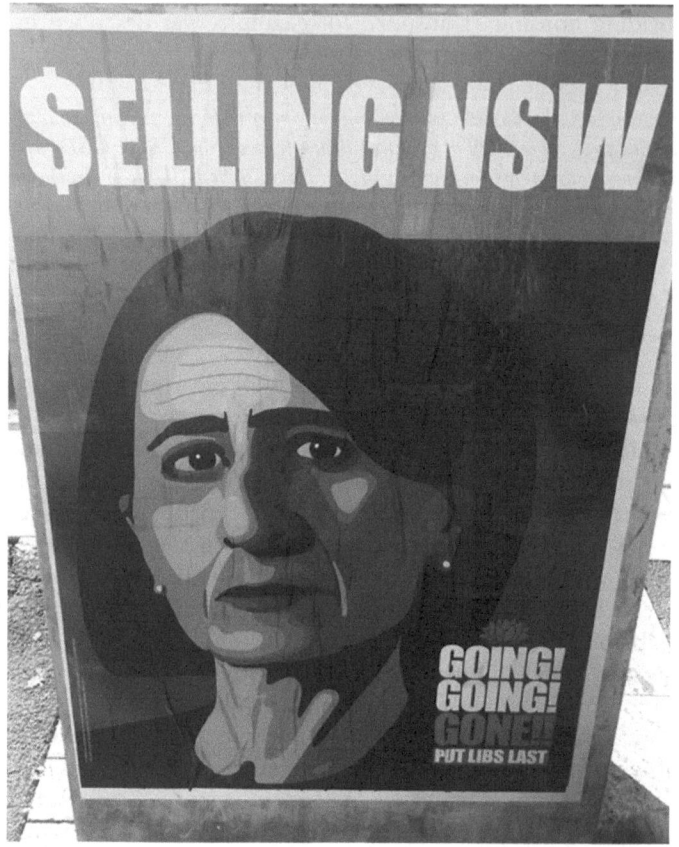

Fig. 7.1 Political poster in the inner west of Sydney during the NSW Election in 2018 (2018, author photo)

via the democratic process. One participant, for instance, explained how in the '80's and '90's the infrastructure sector became dichotomised into being a 'provider' or a 'purchaser'. That separation, however, failed to account for the dual role of government in funding as well as regulating infrastructure. Other participants across the cases raised similar questions about the dual role of **government as both a funder and a regulator**. This became most apparent in the Environmental Assessment where the

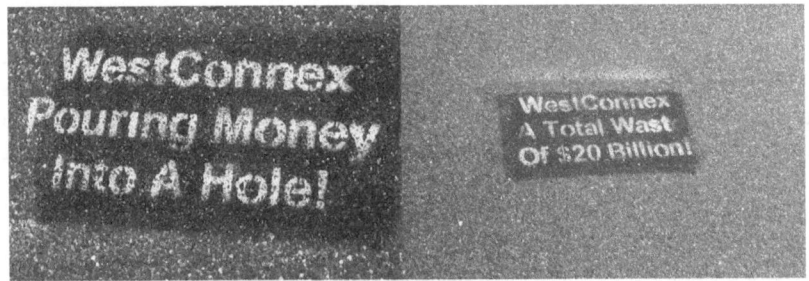

Fig. 7.2 Concerns about the money being spent on the WestConnex road project (2018, author photo)

Planning Department—ultimately the Minister for Planning—assesses and approves projects owned by the Transport Department.

Industry involvement was central to planning given the economic driver mandate of the system. The market loomed so large as a structural force that almost all planning had some kind of private sector focus—who will invest and how, what type of balance of investment is needed, and so forth. The reality is that most infrastructure is built using public money by the private sector. But involving industry was more challenging at a strategic planning level. Public interest concepts like public health are, ultimately, challenging for industry or the private sector to engage with. Terms like 'Outcomes' are used by the private sector, for instance. But, as explained to me during a transport focussed meeting by a partner in a major construction firm, those 'outcomes' are always concerned with the financial bottom line.

The ultimate governance challenge for health is how to represent the public interest. Fortunately, there is a fundamental schism in the infrastructure sector that opens up opportunities for health focussed engagement. The dominance of the market tends to emphasise projects–roads, houses and hospitals—for economic development. Projects bring jobs and are politically nice to sell to the public as they represent delivering tangible 'progress'. The urban and regional planning challenge, I was told, is to shift away from asset driven projects to focus on (re-)investing in existing infrastructural networks. Public health advocates, however, were yet to fully grasp both sides of the infrastructure policy system as opportunities for input and engagement.

Politics, unsurprisingly, plays a fundamental structuring role. Crucially, politics proved motivated by, and accountable to, the wider community. Time and time again I was told how, ultimately, the political decisions that were being made were based on massive dollar figures in response to demands and expectations in the community—housing, jobs, transport, hospitals and health care.

> West Connex in our early conception was about freight access to the port and the airport. So there was a clear commercial imperative. Because you've got a problem, you've got congestion. Our freight network was deficient. It wasn't about people driving cars.
>
> And so you know the idea gets taken over and as it was the case at West Connex it has to because that's what's going to pay for it. And it will be paid for by all those people driving cars, not by trucks. Trucks will contribute but they're 10% of the traffic or whatever.
>
> So you know the idea gets lost by the community expectation; there's a road here, I'm going to drive on it. And so it's very difficult to sort of shift that norm. (Participant, Infrastructure)

These societal expectations, however, were themselves structured within a neoliberal, market dominated frame.

> 'there's a neo-liberal ideology there [in government], there's political donations. And a lot of that comes from the development industry. So where are they getting their money from, how can they *secure power* and maintain power? And that's what politics is often about. So I think that's it, I think we live in a world city with aspirational people. What's most important to a lot of people? Probably their house, probably money, materialism, consumerism, it's the world we live in.' (Participant, strategic planning)

Finally, as this comment introduces, politics intermingled **with power.** Power was so pervasive across this research that I eventually wrote a paper explaining the fundamentals of theories of power for health equity focussed public policy (Harris, Baum et al., 2020a). Power, I experienced and then wrote, was often hidden from view and thus requires a theoretical and critical lens to draw it out and make it visible. There were some observable empirical layers to power as an institutional rule or mandate however. Ultimate power lies with the Premier and Cabinet. Particular portfolios have more power than others: for instance, planning held less power than transport as mentioned. There were battles for power between portfolios and Ministers. These portfolio battles forged siloes in systems. Crossing these silos was challenging and fraught. Integrated planning, for instance, is a good policy mechanism but whether this morphed into actual resources for delivery was essentially a question of how real power was and is shared. The health sector held power but did not wield influence to influence population health through planning. The health system sometimes threw punches into the planning system when hospital (precinct) funding was on the table, but in general tended not to be involved.

Power manifested in battles between groups who were either pro-growth or pro-balance/sustainability. These battles, I discovered, are always occurring at multiple levels of the system—this is the politics in planning. The public, or at least vocal segments of the public who have an overt interest in the Planning system, most often are part of the latter group. The tension between pro-growth and pro-balance was and remains fundamental to how the Planning system is legislated and designed. Generally, the community had a lack of power in negotiations. Processes like Environmental Assessments took power out of the hands of the public and put it into those of experts. There was **overall distrust** between the community and the bureaucratic system exacerbated by technocratic and top-down approach to planning.

IDEAS

Ideas in the political science literature tend to be about the content of policy (Howlett et al., 2009). As I've already shown, ideas are not only represented in policies. They also form the basis of the rules and mandates that structure policy systems. At the same, they overlap closely with actor **interests and values** (Peters, 2019). Ideas can sometimes be clearly expressed and are observable. More often they are implicit, opaque or even hidden.

Health, unsurprisingly, came out as a core idea in the data. While instances of coded content are not my focus here, health was coded more often as an idea. Pre-empting theory, this is because 'health' remains in what political scientists call the 'primordial soup' (or 'garbage can') of ideas vying for policy. Moreover, the **acceptance of health was contested**. Supporters of health tended to unequivocally explain how important health was for the planning system and planners to consider. Others, less supportive or sceptical, either saw it as irrelevant or conceptually too difficult ('too theoretical' has already been discussed).

Framing became an empirical major theme. I often felt that health, public health, planning, cities, etc., are all equally subject to vagaries and whims in policy precisely because they resist any neat definition. They need, in critical realist terms, clarity around boundaries and mechanisms. Planning is essentially characterised by being about a contest of ideas about how a city or region or place should run or be developed. Health is however, in theory, a kaleidoscope of issues that are hard to consider and put on the agenda, even for discussion. At a surface level, the breadth of health issues was seen by many as its undoing as a useful policy concept. The list is long: the determinants of health, health protection, health promotion, environmental health—air, noise and soil quality, active transport, physical activity, liveability. My sense from the research was that, at an empirical layer, health ideas can correspond to the problem that the planning system needs to address. Returning to the point about the two contested sides of infrastructure helps here, as described by one participant:

> At the level of strategic planning and programs of investment and the regulatory decisions saying, "Do we think the *public health* outcomes – other things being equal – would be better or worse if we skewed our investment portfolio one way or another?"
> At the project level – so you've gone from strategy and programs of investment down to individual projects – the public health outcomes will be more tactical but still important. About the volume of emissions concentrated at a particular point, a stack on a tunnel, a level of noise and sleep disruption that might exist around a transport corridor, implications for mental health from having communities disrupted.
>
> (Participant Infra)

This point notwithstanding, ideas are structured by the system in terms of relevance to the problem at hand, and especially the scale of the problem. For instance, EAs in NSW have particular legislative remit to focus in on downstream localities—an infrastructure project can only be assessed for its impact on locations. Any comments about the health of the city, region or planet are out of scope and easily dismissed.

The breadth of health issues is also very contentious because it suggests that health is the central concern over and above other relevant issues (the economy, social, environmental). The technical term for this problematic overreach is 'health imperialism'. 'Health in all policies' is a good example where the framing risks health imperialism (Cairney et al., 2021). As I was told throughout this research, health is a government sector with an already very large, and growing, budget. To suggest that other policy portfolios give up their sovereignty in the name of health risks being a miss-step at the outset when siloes and shoring up of power within sectors is the norm.

An example was an interaction I had when presenting findings on the strategic planning case study back to an interview participant. I was invited back to discuss the findings having produced a draft of our results. That draft essentially supported 'health' being a concern for the whole strategic plan and questioned the 'liveability' focus of that plan. I was pointedly asked 'but what have you got to add?' I was not prepared for the question and flapped around a bit but given my lack of a clear answer I was, I think, dismissed as irrelevant. The experience is seared onto my soul.

In that questioning, however, lies a potential and crucial answer. The empirical evidence from this research shows that considering 'health' for urban and regional planning means accepting that planning systems, like most policy systems, are fundamentally contests over ideas. Each of the case studies centred on this ideational tension and challenge. Ideas were almost always positioned to reinforce particular interests. How health was positioned either supported or challenged these positions. Indeed, the power of health, as well as its weakness, lies in its malleability. A health objective put in place to support legislative reforms that ultimately pushed economic development over and above socio-ecological sustainability is an example (Harris, Kent et al., 2018a, 2018b). But that lack of deep connection to values and interests meant that health objective was easily dismissed when the legislative reforms failed. The lesson was that where health is equivocally or vaguely framed it is often more easily dismissed as irrelevant and less valid.

Equity was raised consistently across the cases. Equity was, surprisingly to me, seen as fundamental to planning. This is likely to be due to sampling—but it is pleasing to note that whether Planning creates or mitigates equity was in the minds of people in positions of real authority. Digging a little deeper into how equity was framed is revealing also. Equity was mostly discussed in terms of spatial inequities. Does transport or greenspace or the built environment exacerbate or alleviate urban inequalities? Or, does the provision of infrastructure allow people on the outer edges of the city to access, by active travel not cars, jobs and services within a reasonable timeframe? Diving deeper into equity and place-making, as I show later in the book, means shifting institutionalised power.

Equity was often conflated with economics, in that economic development would automatically lift up everybody and reduce inequities. This notion of **economic driven equity** was largely unquestioned despite the wealth of evidence to the contrary. The Western Sydney City Deal case drills into this contradiction in detail. Building up a region to be competitive is only part of creating equity. Often the differences within particular regions are harder to shift. For instance, in that original analysis (Harris et al., 2022) we demonstrated how Western Sydney is comparatively disadvantaged to the rest of Sydney. But within the region of Western Sydney, substantial variations exist in populations and the type of infrastructure required to foster better health equity.

Several participants suggested that framing the goal of a **just city** has more impetus for Planners than a healthy city. The argument was that if a city is more just it is more equitable and better equity brings along health benefits. The suggestion made was that equity as justice is attuned with planning politics whereas health is not. One participant went on to explain how the idea of the just city had traction in 'left leaning political circles'. A just city, of course, includes health—especially health equity—but this is an interesting example of how some participants felt an equity frame was more important as the fundamental frame of reference for Planners than a health frame.

> I don't mind a healthy city that's fine, but health on its own is not the healthy city and the more equitable city, the more just city helps that health discussion.
>
> (Participant, Strategic Planning)

The **evidence base for health** revealed contradictory responses from participants. Some participants felt the evidence base was strong and useful. Others felt it was inadequate. Overall, what became apparent was that evidence production and use is very much a technical 'fix' for deeper institutional issues. Almost all participants recognised this:

So you know, the strength of the evidence is critical but it's also the acceptance of the evidence and you find different political perspectives. So I think in most of the circles that I move in there's a broad general acceptance that there are public health outcomes from how we do infrastructure. That's not necessarily reflected in the decisions that are made because there are political pressures on them.

(Participant, Infra)

And another observed how framing the evidence to fit values and interests (ideological preferences) was in fact more important than evidence:

For me I think what's going to be critical is how things are framed. So almost anything that needs to happen in Sydney could be framed as essential for social equity, almost anything that needs to happen could be framed as essential for political viability, and almost anything could be framed up around being essential for global competitiveness. So I think you can make the most of what has to happen fit the ideological preferences of most of the parties... and so we found, for example ... you try and talk to the government around housing density and it's not comfortable talking about housing density because gut feel is that Australians want to live in low density environments. But if you can talk to them about the adverse health outcomes associated with low density sprawl, then all of a sudden they're paying attention in a different way. So I think a lot of this will go to framing.

(Participant, WSCD)

Another example explains the influence of politics on **the utility of evidence**. One participant recalled how evidence supporting the concept of 'the 20 min city' was received by a particularly powerful Federal Minister for Infrastructure. That Minister baulked at 20 min, arguing that this was impossible to deliver and that he would rather 'under promise and over deliver'. So, he added on an extra ten minutes (with car travel). The 'evidence' in policy circles then became known as 'the 30 min city'! Notably the 30 min city subsequently became central to the strategic plans for Greater Sydney led by the GSC, whereas Melbourne's plans have embraced the 20 min concept, and the original idea came from Paris and was 15 minutes.

Evidence is critical but by itself is insufficient to create meaningful institutional change. Indeed because the acceptance of certain types of evidence supports particular interests—quantification of costs and benefits, qualitative data being treated with scepticism, tight risks rather than a full impact causal pathway of determinants, social impacts being under assessed or considered, behaviourism over the structural determinants of health—evidence itself becomes caught up in and perpetuates particular interests and ways of working. Evidence generation and use (or knowledge), it turns out, is presupposed by power relations within institutions. I provide more on this connection between knowledge and power (Flyvbjerg, 1998) through the theoretical lens, but empirically two stark examples suffice at this point.

A community based participant recalled contacting the health department about studying the evidence of the health impact of coal mining projects. The response was that this type of study was not possible because the population affected was not of sufficient size.

> Anyhow, we asked would the government do a study in Singleton but they wrote back and said look, you have to have 25,000 people in two areas to do a study and Singleton only had 23,500. (Participant, Environmental Assessments)

Second was the apparent dismissal in treasury departments of wider externalities for developing business cases for investment decisions:

> But because it's complex and because the links can appear tenuous how that gets reflected in a business case is challenging. So with sustainability broadly, which is consideration of externalities, non-financial impacts, treasury departments, whether it's state or federal, have really struggled with a way to formalise how to address non-financial outcomes in financial decision making. And whether that's environmental outcomes or health outcomes or community outcomes, it's very difficult to get the formalised response which is here are a set of metrics against which we can justify additional investment on the basis of a dividend, a social or a community dividend as opposed to just a straight budgetary dividend. But the private sector is getting increasingly good at that. The way they're doing it is largely by pricing risk.
>
> (Participant, Infrastructure)

Both examples, one local, the other across the whole of society, graphically demonstrate why the holy grail of evidence-informed policy is fraught with institutionalised roadblocks.

Infrastructure became apparent early on as a crucial idea for the planning system, as already mentioned. What became clear in the empirical analysis of infrastructure as an idea was the overt politicisation of the term:

> Your average person doesn't think about infrastructure in that more abstract sense; it's a policy construct. But yes, it's bigger than just your local road or your local bridge. It's grander and, got a bit of a sense of aspiration about it, perhaps. Yes. From a political point-of-view you can be seen to be doing something and the minister gets to make announcements and cut a ribbon at the of it and, "Look what we've done for you."
>
> (Participant, Infrastructure)

Economic growth was the core idea that became a structural mandate, already discussed. Indeed, economic growth acted as the centripetal force behind all the findings. Quite literally everything can be explained in relation to the NSW Planning system being a force to foster economic growth. As noted, there was an inherent and ongoing tension between that economic growth agenda and an agenda to achieve balance with social and environmental concerns. Such language and tensions dominated the discourse in the legislation governing the Planning system and subsequently played out at all levels. Crucially health, equity and related ideas failed, by and large, to capture the collective imagination and manipulate this tension for their advantage.

Climate change was given very little attention. That relative absence had an institutional reason picked up on by several participants in different cases. Essentially, they argued, any reference to climate change ran counter to the political framing of the day which was to ignore the problem as if it was not happening. This was supported by several meetings with politicians I held towards the end of the research, where it was explained to me that the term 'climate change' was not allowed in Parliament. Political parties as well as government departments actively avoided using the term. This purposefully restricted narrative is, thankfully albeit regrettably, changing since the devastating bushfires and resulting smoke in Sydney (see Fig. 7.6) of early 2020. What the data in this research showed, however, was that climate change was caught up in a false either/or argument dichotomy, and resulting **cherry picking of evidence**, around economic development vs sustainability. This was especially apparent in the EA cases—coal mining being the most stark—but occurred across the cases.

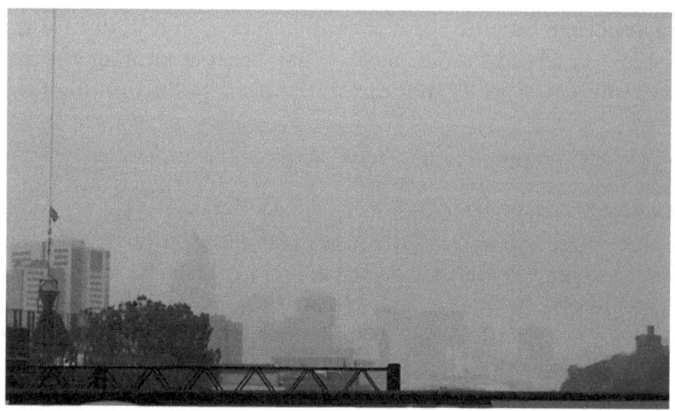

Fig. 7.3 Sydney during the 2020 bushfire crisis

Sustainability was mentioned more often than climate. Sustainability referred mainly to the tension between balanced development—across triple bottom line 'environment, economic and social'—vs an economic growth trumps all agenda. From a population health perspective, it remains puzzling to me that the sustainability angle has yet to be taken up as an idea for healthy planning in NSW. This lack of connection is despite population health impacts and evidence being aligned very closely with sustainable development discourse. Ultimately, the empirical data across the research suggested that whether health is pro-balance or pro-economic growth is something that healthy planning advocates need to take a position on. The lesson from this research about sustainability, and which I go into in much more detail later, is clear. An agnostic position might seem okay in the short term if political expediency is seen as warranted. But if your goal is institutionalisation, being an agnostic is distrusted, soon found out as wanting and easy to ignore.

Finally, **urbanist concepts** abounded across the data. Density, just city, smart cities, infrastructure, agglomeration, place-based, place-making, sprawl, resilience are all examples. What became clear empirically, however, was that health advocates have very little understanding of these crucial concepts that urban and regional planners use (Harris et al., 2016). **Inter-disciplinary discourse deficiency** is a fundamental problem facing 'healthy planning' advocates. Discourse is easy to hide behind as an excuse for not understanding other people's disciplines. As I go on to show later, however, if you want action, discourse is where it all starts.

PROCESSES

Processes proved a useful entry point for many of the practices that open up to deeper institutional analysis. Planning is mostly a practice based on processes (and procedures) that are a mix of formal requirements and informal ways of working. Processes covered a range of activities including developing legislation, use of evidence, budgeting and contracting, the back and forth between bureaucrats and political staffers, developing a strategic plan, environmental assessments to assess a massive infrastructure project, or the creation of networks and coalitions up to and including public private partnerships. Each also acts as an entry point for a deeper understanding of how to create 'healthy planning'.

A process focus emphasised the crucial role that **timing** played across the research and case studies (see also the Policy Cube Chapter 5). Timing is of course essential to the progress of policymaking, even if the structures surrounding policy processes remain relatively unchanged institutionally. Timing, when thought about, becomes the essential construct behind the policy cycle. The **long period** over which this research unfolded, covering 2011–2021, supports Sabatier's observation that around 10 years is necessary to understand a policy (Sabatier, 1998).

I also found that policy change was largely **incremental** over time. Health was off and on the agenda at different points across the life of the research. However, over the course of the research there was discernible recognition of health as an important issue for urban and regional planning processes. Whether that eventuated into health becoming a valued and explicit core concept for the system remains questionable.

Engagement and collaboration were crucial process issues. As mentioned, **engagement with or by the health sector** was on and off and hit and miss in terms of population health. But progress was nevertheless made. Engagement about hospital infrastructure was and remains much more of a consistent focus, although we also found (Harris, Kent et al., 2020b) that good hospital infrastructure planners and administrators were engaged with a broader view of health and expressed frustration with hospitals being the only concern. **Engagement with communities** is a fundamental procedural aspect to urban and regional planning. The politics focus of this research meant I was less interested in the nitty gritty of local engagement, although when community engagement did come up this was invariably a clash of goals and interests. Overall, though, a major finding across the cases—especially Environmental Assessment but also strategic planning—was **the lack of transparency and access to the planning process** for the general public. Perhaps the most dispiriting aspect to the findings was that Environmental Assessment, despite being one of the only regulatory points to engage communities, is not working as a community engagement process. **Intra-government collaboration** was much improved during the research, as mentioned, although questions remain about whether this collaboration leads to meaningful change from a healthy planning perspective or not.

Evidence use is also a process, especially the use of technical evidence within the reality of politics. There was no doubt that much of the evidence presented for policy, especially by the big consultancy firms, erred towards supporting decisions. Consultants explained that the final report or impact statement was the end-product of robust negotiations. Enough to say here at a surface level that **cost benefit analysis** is the most widely used process to filter and generate evidence. From a health perspective, CBA is wanting in its current form (see above comment about evidence). The challenges facing health as an idea in CBA are both its uncertain measurement as a broad issue and the many trade-offs that it encompasses. The most fundamental example of a population health trade-off is infrastructure. Investment in infrastructure is often touted because of its regional benefits 'to the city'. But infrastructure construction and operation will always disrupt the lives of local communities, for better or worse.

CONCLUSION

This chapter has presented the core empirical factors involved in policymaking—actors, structures, ideas and processes—uncovered in my research. The chapter is important not only because of the findings but also as an example of isolating the core empirical dimensions of a complex policy system. The analysis demonstrated how useful the institutional dimension of actors, structures, ideas and processes are in breaking down complex policymaking, with a health lens, into its constituent parts. That said empirical analysis can only ever be the first step in a critical realist piece of healthy public policy analysis. The level of information presented is certainly enough to further understanding, and more than enough to be published as part of a larger body of knowledge. More depth though is required to explain why these various findings came about, and to add a critical lens to practice. Accessing this depth of knowledge and explanation is the subject of the rest of the book. I focus in on theory first, then move to explain the findings across the cases in the light of those theories.

REFERENCES

Cairney, P., Heikkila T., & Wood M. (2019). *Making policy in a complex world.* Cambridge University Press.

Cairney, P., St Denny E., & Mitchell H. (2021). The future of public health policymaking after COVID-19: A qualitative systematic review of lessons from Health in All Policies. *Open Research Europe, 1,* 23.

Flyvbjerg, B. (1998). *Rationality and power: Democracy in practice.* University of Chicago Press.

Giles-Corti, B., Vernez-Moudon, A., Reis, R., Turrell, G., Dannenberg, A. L., Badland, H., Foster, S., Lowe, M., Sallis, J. F., & Stevenson, M. (2016). City planning and population health: A global challenge. *The Lancet, 388*(10062), 2912–2924.

Greiss, G., & Piracha, A. (2021). Post-political planning in Sydney: A turn in the wrong direction. *Australian Planner, 57,* 1–10.

Harris, P., Baum, F., Friel, S., Mackean, T., Schram, A., & Townsend, B. (2020a). A glossary of theories for understanding power and policy for health equity. *Journal of Epidemiology and Community Health, 74*(6), 548–552.

Harris, P., Kent, J., Sainsbury, P., Riley, E., Sharma, N., & Harris, E. (2020b). Healthy urban planning: an institutional policy analysis of strategic planning in Sydney, Australia. *Health Promotion International, 35*(5), 1251.

Harris, P., Riley, E., Dawson, A., Friel, S., & Lawson, K. (2020c). "Stop talking around projects and talk about solutions": Positioning health within infrastructure policy to achieve the sustainable development goals. *Health Policy, 124*(6), 591–598.

Harris, P., Fisher, M., Friel, S., Sainsbury, P., Harris, E., De Leeuw, E., & Baum, F. (2022). City deals and health equity in Sydney Australia. *Health & Place, 73.* https://doi.org/10.1016/j.healthplace.2021.102711

Harris, P., Kent, J., Sainsbury, P., Marie-Thow, A., Baum, F., Friel, S., & McCue, P. (2018a). Creating 'healthy built environment' legislation in Australia; a policy analysis. *Health Promotion International, 33*(6), 1090–1100.

Harris, P., Kent, J., Sainsbury, P., & Thow, A.-M. (2016). Framing health for land-use planning legislation: A qualitative descriptive content analysis. *Social Science & Medicine, 148*, 42–51.

Harris, P., McManus, P., Sainsbury, P., Viliani, F., & Riley, E. (2021). The institutional dynamics behind limited human health considerations in environmental assessments of coal mining projects in New South Wales, Australia. *Environmental Impact Assessment Review, 86*, 106473.

Harris, P., Riley, E., Sainsbury, P., Kent, J., & Baum, F. (2018b). Including health in environmental impact assessments of three mega transport projects in Sydney, Australia: A critical, institutional, analysis. *Environmental Impact Assessment Review, 68*, 109–116.

Haughton, G., & McManus, P. (2019). Participation in postpolitical times. *Journal of the American Planning Association, 85*(3), 321–334.

Hooper, P., Foster, S., Bull, F., Knuiman, M., Christian, H., Timperio, A., Wood, L., Trapp, G., Boruff, B., & Francis, J. J. (2020). Living liveable? RESIDE's evaluation of the "Liveable Neighborhoods" planning policy on the health supportive behaviors and wellbeing of residents in Perth, Western Australia. *Social Science and Medicine Population Health, 10*, 100538.

Howlett, M., Ramesh, M., & Perl, A. (2009). *Studying public policy: Policy cycles and policy sub-systems* (3rd ed.). Oxford University Press.

Hresc, J., Riley, E., & Harris, P. (2018). Mining project's economic impact on local communities, as a social determinant of health: A documentary analysis of environmental impact statements. *Environmental Impact Assessment Review, 72*, 64–70.

Litman, T. (2013). Transportation and public health. *Annual Review of Public Health, 34*, 217–233.

McGreevy, M., Harris, P., Delaney-Crowe, T., Fisher, M., Sainsbury, P., & Baum, F. (2020a). The power of collaborative planning: How a health and planning collaboration facilitated integration of health goals in the 30-year plan for Greater Adelaide. *Urban Policy and Research, 38* (3), 262–275.

McGreevy, M., Harris, P., Delany-Crowe, T., Fisher, M., Sainsbury, P., & Baum, F. (2019). Can health and health equity be advanced by urban planning strategies designed to advance global competitiveness? Lessons from two Australian case studies. *Social Science & Medicine, 242*, 112594.

McManus, P., & Haughton, G. (2020). Sustainability or sustainable infrastructure? Using sustainability discourse to construct a motorway. *Local Environment, 25*(11–12), 985–999.

McManus, P., & Haughton, G. (2021). Fighting to undo a deal: Identifying and resisting the financialization of the WestConnex motorway, Sydney, Australia. *Environment Planning a: Economy Space, 53*(1), 131–149.

NSW Government Office of the Government Architect. (2018). *Better placed*, from https://www.governmentarchitect.nsw.gov.au/policies/better-placed.

Peters, B. G. (2019). *Institutional theory in political science: The new institutionalism.* Edward Elgar Publishing.

Riley, E., Harris, P., Kent, J., Sainsbury, P., Lane, A., & Baum, F. (2017). Including health in environmental assessments of major transport infrastructure projects: A documentary analysis. *International Journal of Health Policy and Management, 7*(2), 144–153.

Riley, E., Sainsbury, P., McManus, P., Colagiuri, R., Viliani, F., Dawson, A., Duncan, E., Stone, Y., Pham, T., & Harris, P. (2019). Including health impacts in environmental impact assessments for three Australian coal-mining projects: a documentary analysis. *Health Promotion International, 35*(3), 449–457.

Robertson, T., McCarthy, A., Jegasothy, E., & Harris, P. (2021). Urban transport infrastructure planning and the public interest: A public health perspective. *Public Health Researchand Practice, 31*(2), 3122108.

Sabatier, P. A. (1998). The advocacy coalition framework: Revisions and relevance for Europe. *Journal of European Public Policy, 5*(1), 98–130.

Sayer, A. (1992). *Method in social science: A realist approach* (2nd ed). Routledge.

Sayer, A. (2000). *Realism and social science.* Sage.

Searle, G., & C. Legacy. (2021). Locating the public interest in mega infrastructure planning: The case of Sydney's WestConnex. *0*(0): 0042098020927835.

Weiss, C. H. (1999). The interface between evaluation and public policy. *Evaluation, 5*(4), 468–486.

CHAPTER 8

Theoretical Comparison: From Theories of the Policy Process to Urban Politics

This chapter presents the results of the theoretical comparison step introduced in Chapter 4. I briefly introduce the step here. I then work through theories of the policy process before spending much of the chapter going deeper into governance and power. I also include a section on taking normative positions in policy and research. The chapter ends by presenting a theoretical proposition about policy goals and governance and power being symbiotic.

A Brief Overview of the Theoretical Comparison Method

Theories, or bodies of theory, are potentially limitless. Accordingly, the core question for a piece of realist research is 'how do I navigate bodies of theory to reinterpret my data?' For this research I took a simple route first, becoming increasingly sophisticated as the research proceeded. The task is to build a theoretical scaffold (Layder, 1998). That analogy is similar to bricolage introduced last chapter. Crucially, theory is compared against the main empirical data for relevance.

I have found the best starting point with any sets of theory is introductions, text or handbooks. As examples, for the research program reported here I variously went to: theories of the policy process (Weible & Sabatier,

2018), political science (Cairney, 2011; Peters, 2019), urban politics (Davies & Imbroscio, 2009; Mossberger et al., 2015) and urban studies (Brenner, 2019; Pierre, 2011).

Rather than go in raw to each body of theory, I had, of course, already gone into detail about the data—presented in Chapter 7—applying the actors, structures, ideas and processes framework. That empirical analysis meant I was already alert to when these bodies of theory might explain something useful and critical about the empirical data. Being systematic helped. Often, I did this in the form of tables to map the core dimensions of those bodies of knowledge against the data driven codes and themes I had developed. I then revisited the critical emerging points from those introductory texts with insights from papers by seminal theorists or reviews. I also read original articles, and where necessary I extended my reading in a snowball manner about particular areas of interest.

The important aspect to this analysis, I found, is to trust instincts while being as systematic as possible. Several critical realist methodologists talk about a lightbulb moment when explanations come together in your head (Danermark et al., 2002; Pawson & Tilley, 1997; Sayer, 2000). That light bulb moment required, for me, deep understanding of the empirical data. The crucial task is to constantly map what theory is telling you about the data. Where theory does not explain the data, it must be let go of as quickly as possible. Otherwise, the process becomes what the critical realist Andrew Sayer (1992, 2000) ominously labels 'empty theorising' for its own sake. The danger of mistakenly going down the wrong theoretical rabbit hole was ever present and, indeed, that distraction away from explaining data occurred frequently. The process was time consuming and those missteps very annoying.

In what follows I present the theoretical comparison journey, I went through for this particular program of research. There were, obviously, lots of theories and disciplines to navigate, in addition to my reviewing of new institutionalism. Essentially, I went through theories of the policy process and on to power and then governance. Disciplines were a mix of political science and urban [studies] politics, with a smattering of supporting public administration and sociology. Urban studies is a discipline that funnels many of these other disciplines while retaining cities as a particular object of attention. New institutionalism, for instance, has been positioned as crucial to urban political theory across both governance and power (Davies & Trounstine, 2012; Lowndes, 2009).

Theories of the Policy Process

Much of my early analysis focussed in on the body of theory known as 'theories of the policy process' (TPP). The aspect of the program this body of theory most helped with was the legislative advocacy case. For the detailed results see (Harris et al., 2018).

Much has been written about TPP. For this phase of the research, I found several sources very useful. Initially I reviewed the (then) most recent compendium[1] of TPP (Sabatier & Weible, 2014). Towards the end of that book Cairney and Heikkila wrote an excellent chapter that systematically compared TPP. I adapted their work—updated in 2018 (Heikkila & Cairney, 2018)—to compare each of the core theories against the essential characteristics of the case-study data, as explained above. Reviewing the theories from this book clarified that some TPP spoke to the data better than other TPP. The theories I ended up focussing on— see Box 8.1—were Multiple Streams Approach (MSA) (Kingdon, 2011; Zahariadis, 2014); Punctuated Equilibrium Theory (PET) (Baumgartner, 2013; Baumgartner et al., 2014); and the Advocacy Coalition Framework (Jenkins-Smith et al., 2014). Having chosen these three from the introductory texts I included concepts from core journal articles focussed on mixing and comparing TPP, for example, see (John, 2003). I also went to the original sources: Kingdon (Kingdon, 2011), a particular book on Punctuated Equilibrium that emphasised decision-making (Jones, 1994), and specific articles by Sabatier (Sabatier, 1988, 1998). I supplemented these core readings with additional articles by the main authors until I felt I had reached theoretical saturation about what they could explain about the data we had collected.

An overview of my take on the core elements of each theory can be found in Box 8.1. Ontologically the three are very close. That understanding of their overlaps demonstrated for me what, in critical realist speak, is 'real' about the policy process. Each clearly finds 'rational behavioural' explanations of policy wanting. Rather, each explains the policymaking process as complex, largely incremental, non-linear, with change taking a long time in the face of entrenched institutional forces. Each provides useful insight to positioning the idea of health onto the

---

[1] The book and that chapter were updated in 2018 version so I suggest going to the newer version.

policy agenda through the actions of multiple stakeholders operating over time and within complex systems.

Box 8.1 Introduction to the theories used for the analysis

The Multiple Streams Approach (MSA) (Kingdon, 2011) focusses on policy choice as 'the combined result of structural forces and cognitive and affective processes that are highly context dependent' (Zahariadis 2014; p. 26). The theory articulates three 'streams', problem, policy and politics, that flow through policy, mostly separately. When these three streams are coupled 'windows of opportunity' for policy influence and change are created. Actors, ideas and structures combine for change to occur over time. Timing, rather than rationality, is crucial. 'Policy entrepreneurs' feature heavily as 'coupling' the three streams.

The advocacy coalition framework (ACF) (Weible and Sabatier 2006) focusses on policy actors' belief systems and policy change involving multiple actors. The theory has two primary units of analysis. One is actors' beliefs, which they are motivated to transfer into policy (Cairney, 2011). The other is the policy subsystem (Jenkins-Smith et al., 2014) where different coalitions, defined by a policy topic (for example land use planning) compete with each other to 'secure outcomes consistent with their beliefs' (p. 200). Actors, the theory suggests, form relatively stable networks, over periods of time, around core beliefs and ideas (Smith & Katikireddi, 2013). Change is categorised by the ACF either as minor or major deviations from the previous policy (Jenkins-Smith et al., 2014). A key enabling factor for change is 'mobilisation by minority coalitions to exploit the event' (ibid., p. 202). Advocacy coalitions then engage in framing contests about these problems.

Punctuated equilibrium theory (PET) (Baumgartner et al., 2014; Jones & Baumgartner 2012) suggests that while policy is characterised by long periods of stability and incrementalism, political processes occasionally produce large scale departures from the past (Baumgartner et al., 2014). There were two core explanatory elements to the theory for the legislative advocacy case. One concerns collective allocation of policymakers' attention and how shifts in attention can, potentially, spawn large changes in policymaking. The other concerns institutions, where policy monopolies form around the dominant image of a policy problem and consequently have the ability to exclude groups who do not support this image.

Despite TPPs obvious value for explaining policymaking, I began at this early point in the research program to question whether TPP might be sufficient for the body of knowledge I was entering into. My reservations[2] essentially concerned depth. Did the explanations generated by TPP go deep enough to explain the data—recalling that the data is concerned with urban and regional planning? Were the theories 'critical' enough? I ended up retaining a core interest in TPP as providing essential insights into policymaking while shifting attention to urban political theory.

Urban Politics: Governance and Power

Two compendiums of Urban Politics (Davies & Imbroscio, 2009; Mossberger et al., 2015) provided the connections to explanations about power and governance that resonated with me as providing necessary explanations for the data. Davies and Imbroscio's coverage rests on the proposition that urban politics is made up of three essential characteristics—power, governance and citizens. Mossberger et al.'s contribution similarly emphasises power and governance as overarching constructs, although not presented in an organising way like Davies and Imbroscio.

Each book has an excellent chapter on New Institutionalism (NI) that also overlaps with a realist emphasis on structure and agency. These two chapters (Davies & Trounstine, 2012; Lowndes, 2009) emphasise that structure and agency are at the heart of governance and power in urban politics[3] Lowndes, for instance, explains NI as driven by concerns with formal and informal rules and conventions and by the way institutions embody value and power relations. And in a point to which I return

[2] Several other authors have actively questioned whether TPP provides sufficient causal depth of synthesis and understanding about policymaking Real-Dato, J. (2009). Mechanisms of policy change: A Proposal for a synthetic explanatory framework. *Journal of Comparative Policy Analysis: Research and Practice*, 11(1), 117–143; van der Heijden, J., Kuhlmann, J., Lindquist, E., & Wellstead, A. (2019). Have policy process scholars embraced causal mechanisms? A review of five popular frameworks. *Public Policy and Administration*: 0952076718814894.

[3] Note at this point the interchanging of authors between urban theory and political science. Davies wrote the chapter on institutionalism in urban politics and the text on urban politics. One of the editors of the Oxford Handbook of Urban Politics is Peter John also wrote one of the seminal critiques of the Big Three TPP (John, 2003). Shortly, I introduce the work of Guy Peters who is an authority on urban governance (Pierre & Peters, 2012) and new institutionalism (Peters, 2019).

repeatedly, she argues that NI rejects structural determinism by emphasising the role of agency as a mechanism *for change* within institutional structures.

With a realist lens, immediate connections to other theorists opened up. This institutional 'structure + agency = change' (see also Peters, 2019) line of reasoning is strongly reminiscent of the work of Pierre Bourdieu (Medvetz & Sallaz, 2018) and the critical realist Margaret Archer (Archer, 1995). Both these social theorists emphasise how structure and agency are embedded within and embody the power dynamics of societies and the (policy) institutions that come to represent those societies. Both structure and agency are distinct and overlapping, but Archer and Bourdieu demonstrate the importance of holding both constructs separate analytically to understand how change comes about. Bourdieu's historical sociological analysis of policy systems in France is particularly good at highlighting how agents are situated within structures but also manipulate those structures to create new structures. That dialectic between structure and agency is demonstrated across my analysis presented in the following chapters.

Both governance and power in urban politics are profoundly influenced by the political economy of globalisation and neoliberalism under the banner of what has come to be known as 'urban competition' (Garcia & Judd, 2012). Urban competition essentially covers competition between cities' within a globalised economy (Jessop, 2002; Jonas & Ward, 2007; Scott & Storper, 2015). The city region approach, following regulation theory, came about in the wake of the transition during the 1970s and 1980s from Fordist-Keynesian capital accumulation and welfare state provision to 'flexible accumulation' and loosening of regulation to emphasise market rationality, deregulation and privatisation (Badcock, 2014). I come back to that fundamental shift from welfarism to market rationality as a core explanation for why the data showed that health equity struggled for a foothold in Planning policy.

Several mechanisms sit behind the City as the 'centres of economic production and exchange' (Scott & Storper, 2015). One, agglomeration, is a policy goal that concerns the spatial clustering of divisions of labour, sharing urban services as public goods, matching people and jobs, and stimulating innovation through formal and informal information flows (Scott & Storper, 2015). Another, urban managerialism, reflects Keynesian economics being overtaken by 'new urban entrepreneurialism' in response to the declining powers of states to control the out-flow of capital to multinationals, 'to maximise the attractiveness of the local site [the city region] as a lure for capitalist development' (Harvey, 1989). Put simply, global city region competition forced city policymakers to become entrepreneurial (Garcia & Judd, 2012). In terms of governance arrangements, the restructuring of state power under the challenges of neoliberalism and globalisation means that cities and regions must restructure their institutional frameworks and policy choices (Davies & Imbroscio, 2009; Garcia & Judd, 2012; McCann, 2017). These urban political economy dynamics surround, indeed condition, governance and power.

This 'city region' thesis is not without its detractors. As noted in Chapter 3 (when I introduced the debate in urban studies about realism vs Marxism), there has been a long-standing debate in urban studies challenging the 'totalising' discourse of cities being in thrall to global forces of competition (Brenner, 2019; Harvey, 1987). What falls out of those criticisms is the need for a *relational* view of city policy and urban planning (Healey, 2006b). A relational view sees urban spaces and places and multi-layered, connected up to global policy systems and down into local communities. Brenner (2019) explains the relational approach via seminal urbanist Henri Le Febvre's analogy of a millefeuille, the dessert made up of 'a thousand layers'.

Coming full circle back to the health literature[4] taking a relational view has been championed in the health equity literature (Corburn, 2017). Building on the work of Healey (2006b), Corburn argues that a relational view of place is necessary to bring health equity into urban policy. That relational view, Corburn argues, requires attending to urban politics, governance and power (and empowerment). Recalling my introduction to the evidence on place-making for health equity in Chapter 2, the relational view is covered by a strong evidence base linking people—'compositional characteristics'—with the environment—'context' (Arcaya et al., 2016; Bambra, 2016; Cummins et al., 2007). Our original paper on the Western Sydney City Deal goes into that relational evidence and political reality in great detail (Harris et al., 2022).

But what makes structure and agency fire in the type of data I had collected? As noted in earlier chapters, across the analysis I was pursuing I knew that power was at the core of the analysis. So, it was unsurprising to

---

[4] I referred to Jason Corburn's work earlier in the book (Chapter 2) with reference to health cities and the politics of urban healthy public policy.

me that power was similarly central to urban political theory. Governance soon became as important as power. In reality of course governance and power intertwine, as follows.

Governance in urban politics—as in political science and public administration—is essentially the blurring of traditional relationships, boundaries and accountabilities between networks of public, private and civil actors (McCann, 2017). Government is the principle facilitator of governance arrangements and 'urban bureaucrats' are essentially mediators and networkers, securing action through participation and partnerships (Brandtner et al., 2017; Healey et al., 2002a, b). In the modern era, post-Fordist, model of accumulation, cities' institutional governance arrangements revolve around working across layers of government and actors outside of government (Jessop, 2002). And in a crucial line of reasoning for my research, governance cultures in cities have been shown to both follow an institutional path dependency and are dynamic and innovative (Garcia & Judd, 2012). Path dependencies are essentially the historical baggage that institutions carry with them, and which mean policymaking systems tend to be oriented towards stasis or maintenance of existing power structures via particular regimes of powerful actors.[5] These dependencies refer to structured, institutionalised, ways of making policy that are rusted on and tough to shift (Koch, 2013). In urban studies for instance,

> overarching conditions of political authority and power leave deep traces on urban development … that define the scope of policy, planning activities, the spatial functioning of the 'urban land' nexus, and local politics. (Scott & Storper, 2015) (p. 11)

Change is therefore extremely hard to come by because of these historically embedded ways of working. Nevertheless, both political science and urban studies assert institutional governance change as the lynchpin behind all policy work—maintaining the status quo in the face of challenges, or mounting challenges to the status quo (Healey, 2006a;

---

[5] TPP are very strong on path dependencies, where the big three—ACF, PET and multiple streams—all rest on the notion that policy subsystems are very hard to change because of path dependencies and require significant and strategic action by agents and actors to create change or, as in the name given to PET, 'punctuate the equilibrium'.

Immergut, 2006; Steele, 2011). From a healthy public policy perspective, the challenge is similarly institutional (Harris et al., 2020), i.e. has the planning system taken on health as a core policy value and goal as well as implemented actions to achieve that goal and cement that value throughout the system?

Governance, as a mix of path dependency on the one hand and strategy for innovation on the other, is crucial for Healthy Public Policy advocates to understand. For instance, in a set of papers that gave me a 'lightbulb' moment, McGuirk (2005, 2007) explains strategic planning in Sydney as driven by a complex web of motivations including social justice, global competitiveness and political legitimacy. Mc Guirk positions Sydney's metropolitan plans as institutional compromises, largely framed through an economic lens, responding to multiple demands on the State from communities and industry for differing forms of infrastructure upgrades to manage urban problems. During the analysis of case studies that follows in the next chapters, the many and multiple motivations by actors who also hold different levels of power to create and influence change comes through strongly. Using theory, I show how policymakers are often working at different points in the urban and regional policy system, often holding differing levels of power to change (or maintain) ways of making policy.

Normative Positioning: What 'Should' Happen

I want here to take a brief detour into why theory itself needs to be challenged when searching for critical explanations about empirical data. I introduced the normative dimension to policy (and research) in the first part of the book. Specifically in Chapter 4 I called for critical lens on the use of theory in science. Here I bring that cautionary take about theoretical positions into my analysis as a distinct category. I do this by first taking a normative lens to urban political theory, and then applying that normative critique to theories of urban governance. As I explained in Chapter 3, all research and theory has a normative (value positions about what should happen) base which ought to be critiqued if we want to use those theories to explain data. In the urban politics literature, for instance, Pierre and Peters conclude their chapter with the observation that 'at some stage or another, assessing governance arrangements becomes almost impossible without some normative benchmarks' (p. 84).

One of the criticisms that can be levelled at urban studies is that the much of the theorising and research about urban politics is normatively driven by unwavering support of city region competition driven by market mechanisms. The preference for the Competitive City over and above other normative approaches to what urban politics could be, for instance, the Just City, is questionable when the result is greater social inequalities (Garcia & Judd, 2012; Pill, 2021). For example, entrepreneurial approaches to government can be legitimated in contexts like the US but come with in-built inequity: 'winners being sharply divided from losers' and an ambiguous state autonomy from private interests (p 494; Garcia & Judd, 2012). Indeed, the arguable initiator of urban governance, regime theory (Stone, 2005) was US based. Regime theory went on to inspire analysis subsequently shown to have a (normative) tendency towards neoliberalism. Economically driven regimes were seen as successful, while regimes structured around environmental or social agendas less so as these were more difficult to mobilise resources for and to sustain (Mossberger, 2009; Sapotichne & Jones, 2012). From a healthy public policy perspective, this normative critique is crucial; creativity and innovation to enhance intra-urban competition are fundamentally challenged by a social equity critique (De Leeuw et al., 2021). I return to these normative points and supporting literature in the final chapter of the book.

Taking on normative positions is not just empty theoretical critique. It turns out that when we accept that urban politics is normative, we begin to see how urban policy practice manifests itself. Stating an urban policy position about city region competitiveness provides theorists and policymakers with a fundamental goal about what cities should strive to become. Such goals, the urban politics literature shows, then structure the subsequent composition of governance to achieve those goals (Pierre, 1999, 2011). This crucial explanatory proposition for the research is developed further in the next section.

Goals and Objectives Meet Governance Composition

In one of the best chapters on urban governance (Pierre & Peters, 2012), Pierre—whose substantive area is local governance—and Peters—an institutionalist—explain why the connection between governance composition and policy objectives is crucial. Their main point is that because governance networks are composed by a constellation of actors sharing the same basic interests and objectives, the composition of governance arrangements and policy objectives are 'defined in one and the same process' (p. 81). I show in the next chapters how these governance arrangements are defined by discursive narratives that form around different planning objectives, mostly within an economic growth and/or market driven narrative. In practice, governance 'success', because of the inevitable mix of agencies and actors with different agendas and ways of working, requires establishing ongoing mechanisms for inter-agency checks and balances to manage ever present risks of failure (Jessop, 1998; Stoker, 1998). In a point where structure meets agency as part of governance, Pierre and Peters argue that positive change can occur with the right mix of political leadership and accountability.

Goals, then, matter because they intertwine with governance through power. Urban governance aimed at shoring up global competition may also shore up existing uneven power relations rather that delivering on promises of greater democracy and grass roots empowerment (Swyngedouw, 2005). The top down, Competitive City approach to urban governance has been subject to sustained critique that argues how localised, bottom up strategies are also necessary especially where social justice and equity are concerned (McCann, 2017). Concerning infrastructure, for example, David Harvey's seminal urban political analysis cautioned that while infrastructure investments can benefit whole regions they tend instead to favour local 'coalitions of property developers and financiers' (Harvey, 1989). The ultimate governance challenge facing cities, such political economic theories state, is the balance between fostering private investment, integrating the business community into collectively defined activities, while asserting just enough regulatory or policy control that business does not relocate because of regulatory constraints (Pierre & Peters, 2012).

Many of these core ideas about governance were embodied in Curtis Stone's seminal Urban Regime Theory (Stone, 2005). Regime theory ultimately morphed into theories of urban governance and power and their application in local contexts (Garcia & Judd, 2012; Sapotichne & Jones, 2012). The architect of urban regime theory, Clarence Stone, has written an interesting overview of power analysis in urban studies (Stone, 2015).

From this premise he suggests that power reinforces the core characteristics of urban governance, intertwined with interests and goals:

- *Policy directions* are essential. Adding fluidity (and time) to how policy goals influence and direct policy, Stone explains that it is the trajectory of policy that is important because power is not static.
- *Scope of agency* focusses on how *choices* come about in varying scopes—e.g. long or short, narrow or broad. Agency, he argues, is concerned with agendas, and those agendas, rather than isolated decisions, are the 'major landmarks for policy direction'. Stone thus accepts that agendas, through agency, can structure policymaking.
- *Decision processes* are as important as substantive issues.
- *Coalition building*[6] is crucial as opposed to domination and suppression. The worthwhile premise for this emphasis is noted by Stone because the original faces of power theory (Lukes, 2005) focussed solely on suppression, or 'power over', via structural determinism (see also Harris et al., 2020).
- *Powerlessness brought about by social change.* Essentially, Stone argues that some in the community are left out as broad, impersonal, policy changes unfold.

Governance, urban regimes usefully have been defined as containing the following dimensions—shown in Box 8.2. Each of these dimensions is similar to how theorists in the public administration literature have characterised governance frameworks and regimes (Jessop, 1998; Stoker, 1998).[7] The items challenged by urban governance theory which involves moving away from static 'horizontal' or 'vertical' regimes which are characteristic of the 'new public management' approaches to policy (Kjaer, 2009). Instead, 'new urban governance' is network based (Kjaer, 2009) and flexible over time. That flexibility is necessary considering the ever present path dependencies that are inevitable in policy and the dynamism required for change to eventuate (Healey, 2006b; Healey et al., 2002a, b; Pierre & Peters, 2012). The ultimate institutional question remains,

---

[6] Sabatier's Advocacy Coalition Framework rests on the same premise.

[7] Jessop (1998)—whose disciplinary bases cover a mix of critical realism, urban political science, statism and public administration—argues for a mix of horizontal and vertical governance. His concept 'Heterarchical governance' is similar to what political scientists have recently been unpacking as 'policy-centric' governance for understanding policymaking in a complex world (Cairney, P., Heikkila, T., & Wood, M. [2019]. *Making policy in a complex world*. Cambridge University Press.

however, whether flexible regimes take on new voices and new ideas that necessarily challenge the rusted on status quo (Healey et al., 2002a, b).

Box 8.2 Core governance characteristics of urban regimes (Mossberger & Stoker, 2001; Stone, 2005)
- Identifiable policy agendas related to the composition of partners in the coalition.
- Partners from government and nongovernment sources, requiring but not limited to business participation.
- Resources, often from disparate sources, to support collaboration to pursue the agenda and accomplish tasks.
- Long standing schemes of cooperation among members.

This may well be one of these points in this book to ask 'what has this got to do health?' A lot, it turns out. Navigating governance and power means articulating what is needed to position and maintain health-related ideas in public policy.

Pierre and Peters's (2012) proposition is that governance processes and policy objectives are inherently intertwined and mutually reinforcing over time. Inserting 'health' focussed objectives and then delivering on them in practice requires supportive governance regimes. For those, who are interested in how governance matters for healthy public policy I suggest reviewing an excellent paper about governance for intersectoral health focussed policy action (De Leeuw, 2017). De Leeuw builds on political science theory to show how governance for health equity is multi-layered (and relational, and institutional). Just like Pierre and Peters' proposition that goals define governance and governance defines goals, De Leeuw shows how institutionalising health equity through health in all policies requires governance built on goals, objectives and then leadership, capacity and resources across sectors to achieve those goals and objectives.

Moving back into urban studies, an important piece of the governance puzzle within my research program came from urban governance theorising. Pierre (1999, 2011) provides an archetypal analytic framework that presupposes his thesis that goals and governance are symbiotic. He suggests various 'defining characteristics of urban policy and commensurate models of urban governance'. His analysis is shown in Table 8.1.

Table 8.1   Pierre's urban governance framework (Pierre, 1999, 2011)

	Managerial	Corporatist	Pro-growth	Welfare
Key evaluative criterion	Efficiency	Participation	Growth	Equity
Policy objectives	Efficiency	Distribution	Growth	Redistribution
Policy style	Pragmatic	Ideological	Pragmatic	Ideological
Nature of political exchange	Consensus	Conflict	Consensus	Conflict
Nature of public-private exchange	Competitive	Concerted	Interactive	Restrictive
Local state-citizen relationship	Exclusive	Inclusive	Exclusive	Inclusive
Primary contingency	Professionals	Civic leaders	Business	The state
Key instruments	Contracts	Deliberations	Partnerships	Networks
Pattern of subordination	Positive	Negative	Positive	Negative

What the data in my research suggests is that almost all of the urban and regional policy system in NSW is geared towards the 'Pro-growth' model of urban governance. As you will see in the rest of this section, this normative emphasis then played out across the cases in very similar ways to those that Pierre's framework suggests. I then mapped this onto the work of Kjaer (2009), who as noted earlier differentiates top down, new public management governance approaches as ineffective compared to the new urban governance mix of horizontal and vertical networks (just as do De Leeuw, 2017, Jessop, 1998; Stoker, 1998).

This seemingly crucial piece to the theoretical puzzle that the data presented is a good example of needing to think critically about the normative theoretical constructs being brought to bear in a piece of analysis. Pierre (1999), when coming up with this very useful heuristic framework, did so from a normative position about what is best for urban governance. His value position is given away in his explanation of the welfare column, which he dismisses as 'anticapitalistic' and 'needy for private investment but least geared for attracting such investment' (1999, p. 387). As I show in later chapters, this type of archetypal pitching based on normative positions is overly simplistic and may perpetuate problems inherent in urban political practice. Shake it up a bit and reality is far more complex, especially, when a relational view of health and place is taken.

SUMMARY

In summary, this chapter navigated theories of the policy process and urban politics that help to explain the empirical data presented in the previous chapter. When comparing theories against the data, it became clear that governance and power, provided vital explanatory depth. Those explanations covered everything from context—post-fordist global accumulation—to structures—the power of institutional path dependency opening up and closing opportunities for change—to agency—sharing of power through governance to achieve shared interests. I presented a core proposition, that policy goals, which is normative 'what should happen' positions, are in a symbiotic power laden relationship with governance regimes. Healthy public policy, thus, requires being involved in and manipulating governance regimes.

REFERENCES

Arcaya, M. C., Tucker-Seeley, R. D., Kim, R., Schnake-Mahl, A., So, M., & Subramanian, S. (2016). Research on neighborhood effects on health in the United States: A systematic review of study characteristics. *Social Science & Medicine, 168*, 16–29.

Archer, M. S. (1995). *Realist social theory: The morphogenetic approach.* Cambridge University Press.

Badcock, B. (2014). *Making sense of cities: A geographical survey.* Routledge.

Bambra, C. (2016). *Health divides: Where you live can kill you.* Policy Press.

Baumgartner, F. R., Jones, B. D., & Mortensen, P. B. (2014). Punctuated equilibrium theory: Explaining stability and change in public policymaking. In C. Weible & P. Sabatier (Eds.), *Theories of the policy process* (pp. 59–103).

Brandtner, C., Höllerer, M. A., Meyer, R. E., & Kornberger, M. (2017). Enacting governance through strategy: A comparative study of governance configurations in Sydney and Vienna. *Urban Studies, 54*(5), 1075–1091.

Brenner, N. (2019). *New urban spaces: Urban theory and the scale question.* Oxford University Press.

Cairney, P. (2011). *Understanding public policy: Theories and issues.* Palgrave Macmillan.

Cairney, P., Heikkila, T., & Wood, M. (2019). *Making policy in a complex world.* Cambridge University Press.

Corburn, J. (2017). Urban place and health equity: Critical issues and practices. *International Journal of Environmental Research and Public Health, 14*(2), 117.

Cummins, S., Curtis, S., Diez-Roux, A. V., & Macintyre, S. (2007). Under-standing and representing 'place'in health research: a relational approach. *Social Science & Medicine, 65*(9), 1825–1838.

Danermark, B., Ekstrom, L., Jakobsen, L., & Karlsson, J. C. (2002). *Explaining society: Critical realism and the social sciences.* Routledge.

Davies, J. S., & Imbroscio, D. L. (2009). *Theories of urban politics.* Sage.

Davies, J. S., & Trounstine J. (2012a). Urban politics and the new institution-alism. In K. Mossberger, S. E. Clarke, & P. John (Eds.), *The Oxford handbook of urban politics* (pp. 51–70).

De Leeuw, E. (2017). Engagement of sectors other than health in integrated health governance, policy, and action. *Annual Review of Public Health, 38*(1), 329–349.

De Leeuw, E., Harris, P., Kim, J., & Yashadhana, A. (2021, December). A health political science for health promotion. *Global Health Promotion, 28*(4), 17–25.

Garcia, M., & Judd, D. R. (2012). Competitive cities. In S. E. Clarke, P. John, & K. Mossberger (Eds.), *The Oxford handbook of urban politics* (p. 486).

Harris, P., Fisher, M., Friel, S., Sainsbury, P., Harris, E., De Leeuw, E., & Baum, F. (2022). City deals and health equity in Sydney, Australia. *Health & Place, 73.*

Harris, P., Kent, J., Sainsbury, P., Marie-Thow, A., Baum, F., Friel, S., & McCue, P. (2018). Creating 'healthy built environment' legislation in Australia; A policy analysis. *Health promotion international, 33*(6), 1090–1100.

Harris, P., Kent, J., Sainsbury, P., Riley, E., Sharma, N., & Harris, E. (2020). Healthy urban planning: an institutional policy analysis of strategic planning in Sydney, Australia. *Health Promotion International, 35*(5), 1251.

Harvey, D. (1987). Reconsidering social theory: A debate. *Environment and Planning D: Society and Space, 5*(4), 367–434.

Harvey, D. (1989). From managerialism to entrepreneurialism: The transforma-tion in urban governance in late capitalism. *Geografiska Annaler: Series B, Human Geography, 71*(1), 3–17.

Healey, P. (2006a). Transforming governance: Challenges of institutional adap-tation and a new politics of space. *European Planning Studies, 14*(3), 299–320.

Healey, P. (2006b). *Urban complexity and spatial strategies: Towards a relational planning for our times.* Routledge.

Healey, P., Cars, G., Madanipour, A., & De Magalhaes, C. (2002a). Trans-forming governance, institutionalist analysis and institutional capacity. In G. Cars, P. Healey, A., Madanipour, & C. De Magalhães (Eds.), *Urban governance, institutional capacity and social milieux* (pp. 20–42). Routledge.

Healey, P., Cars, G., Madanipour, A., & de Magalhães, C. (2002b). Urban governance capacity in complex societies: challenges of institutional adaptation. In G. Cars, P. Healey, A., Madanipour, & C. De Magalhães (Eds.), *Urban governance, institutional capacity and social milieux* (pp. 204–225).

Heikkila, T., & Cairney, P. (2018). *Comparison of theories of the policy process* (pp. 301–327). Routledge.

Immergut, E. M. (2006). *Historical-institutionalism in political science and the problem of change* (pp. 237–259). Springer.

Jenkins-Smith, H., Nohrstedt, D., Weible, C., & Sabatier, P. (2014). The advocacy coalition framework: Foundations, evolution, and ongoing research. In P. Sabatier & C. Weible (Eds.), *Theories of the policy process*. Routledge.

Jessop, B. (1998). The rise of governance and the risks of failure: The case of economic development. *International Social Science Journal, 50*(155), 29–45.

Jessop, B. (2002). Liberalism, neoliberalism, and urban governance: A state–theoretical perspective. *Antipode, 34*(3), 452–472.

John, P. (2003). Is there life after policy streams, advocacy coalitions, and punctuations: Using evolutionary theory to explain policy change? *Policy Studies Journal, 31*(4), 481–498.

Jonas, A. E., & Ward, K. (2007). Introduction to a debate on city-regions: New geographies of governance, democracy and social reproduction. *International Journal of Urban and Regional Research, 31*(1), 169–178.

Jones, B. D. (1994). *Reconceiving decision-making in democratic politics: Attention, choice, and public policy*. University of Chicago Press.

Jones, B. D., & Baumgartner, F. R. (2012). From there to here: Punctuated equilibrium to the general punctuation thesis to a theory of government information processing. *Policy Studies Journal, 40*(1), 1–20.

Kingdon, J. W. (2011). *Agendas, Alternatives, and Public Policies* (3rd Ed.). Ill, Pearson Education Inc.

Kjær, A. M. (2009). Governance and the urban bureaucracy. In J. S. Davies & D. L. Imbroscio (Eds.), *Theories of urban politics* (pp. 137–152). Sage.

Koch, P. (2013). Overestimating the shift from government to governance: Evidence from Swiss metropolitan areas. *Governance, 26*(3), 397–423.

Layder, D. (1998). *Sociological practice: Linking theory and social research*. Sage Publications.

Lowndes, V. (2009). New institutionalism and urban politics. *Theories of Urban Politics, 2*, 91–105.

Lukes, S. (2005). *Power: A radical view*. Palgrave Macmillan.

McCann, E. (2017). Governing urbanism: Urban governance studies 1.0, 2.0 and beyond. *Urban Studies, 54*(2), 312–326.

McGuirk, P. (2005). Neoliberalist planning? Re-thinking and re-casting Sydney's metropolitan planning. *Geographical Research, 43*(1), 59–70.

McGuirk, P. (2007). The political construction of the city-region: Notes from Sydney. *International Journal of Urban and Regional Research, 31*(1), 179–187.

Medvetz, T., & Sallaz, J. J. (2018). *The Oxford handbook of Pierre Bourdieu.* Oxford University Press.

Mossberger, K. (2009). Urban regime analysis. *Theories of Urban Politics, 2,* 40–54.

Mossberger, K., Clarke, S. E., & John, P. (2015). *The Oxford handbook of urban politics.* Oxford University Press.

Mossberger, K., & Stoker, G. (2001). The evolution of urban regime theory: The challenge of conceptualization. *Urban Affairs Review, 36*(6), 810–835.

Pawson, R., & Tilley, N. (1997). *Realistic evaluation.* Sage Publications Ltd.

Peters, B. G. (2019). *Institutional theory in political science: The new institutionalism.* Edward Elgar Publishing.

Pierre, J. (1999). Models of urban governance: The institutional dimension of urban politics. *Journal of Urban Affairs Review, 34*(3), 372–396.

Pierre, J. (2011). *The politics of urban governance.* Palgrave Macmillan.

Pierre, J., & Peters, B. G. (2012). Urban governance. In K. Mossberger, S. E. Clarke, & P. John (Eds.), *The Oxford handbook of urban politics.*

Pill, M. (2021). *Governing cities: Politics and policy.* Springer.

Real-Dato, J. (2009). Mechanisms of policy change: A proposal for a synthetic explanatory framework. *Journal of Comparative Policy Analysis: Research and Practice, 11*(1), 117–143.

Sabatier, P. A. (1988). An advocacy coalition framework of policy change and the role of policy-oriented learning therein. *Policy Sciences, 21*(2), 129–168.

Sabatier, P. A. (1998). The advocacy coalition framework: Revisions and relevance for Europe. *Journal of European Public Policy, 5*(1), 98–130.

Sabatier, P. A., & Weible, C. (2014). *Theories of the policy process.* Westview Press.

Sapotichne, J., & Jones, B. D. (2012). *Setting city agendas: Power and policy change.* Oxford University Press.

Sayer, A. (1992). *Method in social science: A realist approach* (2nd ed.). Routledge.

Sayer, A. (2000). *Realism and social science.* Sage Publications.

Scott, A. J., & Storper, M. (2015). The nature of cities: The scope and limits of urban theory. *International Journal of Urban and Regional Research, 39*(1), 1–15.

Smith, K. E., & Katikireddi, S. V. (2013). A glossary of theories for understanding policymaking. *Journal of Epidemiology and Community Health, 67*(2), 198–202.

Steele, W. (2011). Strategy-making for sustainability: An institutional learning approach to transformative planning practice. *Planning Theory & Practice, 12*(2), 205–221.

Stoker, G. (1998). Governance as theory: Five propositions. *International Social Science Journal, 50*(155), 17–28.

Stone, C. N. (2005). Looking back to look forward: Reflections on urban regime analysis. *Urban Affairs Review, 40*(3), 309–341.

Stone, C. N. (2015). Power. In E. Mossberger, S. Clarke & J. Peter (Eds.), *Oxford handbook of urban politics*. Oxford University Press.

Swyngedouw, E. (2005). Governance innovation and the citizen: The Janus face of governance-beyond-the-state. *Urban Studies, 42*(11), 1991–2006.

van der Heijden, J., Kuhlmann, J., Lindquist, E., & Wellstead, A. (2019). Have policy process scholars embraced causal mechanisms? A review of five popular frameworks. *Public Policy and Administration*. 0952076718814894.

Weible, C. M., & Sabatier, P. (2018). *Theories of the policy process*. Routlege.

Zahariadis, N. (2014). Ambiguity and multiple streams. In P. Sabatier & C. Weible (Eds.), *Theories of the policy process* (pp. 25–58). Westview Press.

Section 2: Healthy Planning Through the Lens of Governance and Power

This section of the book presents revised and deepened explanations of the empirical data collected across the research. The section corresponds to the retroductive/abductive analysis and 'recontextualisation' phases of critical realist research introduced in Part I (Chapter 4). The findings are structured against the core categories introduced in the previous chapter. The analysis is driven by the core theories introduced in that chapter. As the analysis unfolds, I add additional theoretical insights from other supporting literature.

What is presented is a theoretical explanation of healthy urban and regional planning in Sydney and surrounding regions from 2011 to 2021. At the heart of that explanation is Pierre and Peters' (2012) proposition, introduced last chapter, that policy objectives governance and power are intertwined and mutually reinforcing. I artificially tease them apart here. Governance comes first and then power. I then add, also introduced last chapter, normative analysis for what I think is required to progress 'healthy planning' in the light of the research findings. I include a 'post-script' that briefly sums up the work and situates it back into a realist methodology.

CHAPTER 9

Governance

This chapter focusses attention on governance. The chapter develops the proposition that a system goal of economic capital is fundamental to the governance frameworks and regimes established across the planning system to progress that goal. Health, I show, struggled when health focussed advocates, experts or stakeholders were absent from the governance table.

I start with the strategic end of the system, where I focus on how the government as primary stakeholder struggled to shift to a new form of urban governance that is flexible and accommodates health as a broad concept. I then shift to Environmental Assessments of major infrastructure projects, finding these processes were wanting from public health perspective in terms of governance as well as content. Third, I turn to the Western Sydney City Deal to show how new ideas about governance were opportunities for a health agenda but struggled for meaningful institutional change.

STRATEGIC PLANNING: STUCK IN THE NEW PUBLIC MANAGEMENT RATHER THAN FLEXIBLE GOVERNANCE

We were lucky enough to capture two instances of strategic planning (Harris, Kent et al., 2020). One of these was in 2013 and the next was five

© The Author(s), under exclusive license to Springer Nature
Switzerland AG 2022
P. Harris, *Illuminating Policy for Health*, Palgrave Studies
in Public Health Policy Research,
https://doi.org/10.1007/978-3-031-13199-8_9

years later, in 2018. The first plan, A Plan for Growing Sydney (APGS) was explained as reflecting the government's economic growth agenda to be implemented through central government driven system where resources, ideas and decisions flow from the top to eventually benefit lower and local levels. We analysed the data about APGS against Kjaer's (2009, p. 140) comparison of the assumptions under public management (old and new) and urban governance theory. Our analysis showed that APGS conformed to new public management assumptions rather than new urban governance. Essentially, the government positioned the plan as providing the enabling environment for the market rather than as facilitator of network governance with multiple stakeholders. APGS came to be dominated by the siloed nature of policymaking in NSW and the relative lack of power of the Department of Planning within this context, including a relatively limited budget. The setting of targets or actions that required the buy in and funds of other sectors was inevitably problematic. APGS consequently suffered from a distinct lack of a mechanism or mandate to implement, such that it was seen as a plan with no accountability for delivery. Health, for instance, was given its moment in the sun in the APGS, directly influenced by renewed interest in the idea because of the advocacy around the failed 2011–2013 legislative reforms. But despite being a core goal, no health focussed targets or implementation strategies were developed.

Against Kjaer's (2009) framework of urban policy approaches, the discourse of the later tranche of 2018 district plans was firmly in the mode of new urban governance—collaboration, consensus and facilitation, to achieve their more flexible ESD objectives. Interviewees consistently positioned both the District Plans and the Greater Sydney Commission (GSC) as instruments to facilitate governance across the siloed workings of different agencies (including the private sector). As one interviewee described it, the GSC and the plans were seen as a 'new opportunity' for coordinating a vision for the city. However, our analysis showed that the GSC faced an uphill struggle to shift actual—path dependent, a concept defined in detail last chapter—ways of working away from new public management to networked governance. Although described by one interviewee as a good example of 'modern collaborative thinking', the new concept of governance which the GSC embodied was still described as existing without meaningful regulatory mechanisms to anchor its plans into the system of governance in NSW. This, participants explained, risked the District Plans having very little authority to ensure the land use outcomes they envisioned were delivered.

The later District plans included, in line with the legislated function of the GSC (NSW Government, 2015), a primary goal to deliver infrastructure (along with goals of liveability, productivity and sustainability). That infrastructure mandate given to the GSC was potentially discordant with the infrastructure investment and delivery program of the NSW state government. State infrastructure investment decisions, we were told, including decisions on specific health infrastructure, occur in the state's Cabinet on the advice from Treasury and override both the statutory responsibilities and the geographical Greater Sydney remit of the GSC. There are, however, some opportunities for influence. For example, state agencies, including Health, are required to develop Capital Investment Plans that provide a summary of total physical asset commitments over a 10-year timeframe. The GSC, we showed, had opportunity to influence these plans as capital investment funding is committed annually. Health, however, tends to be positioned in these decisions as hospital infrastructure. By dangling the allure of infrastructure funding attached to health precincts, the GSC and the District Plans activated competition between the local level authorities responsible for health (known in NSW as Local Health Districts), largely around funding for hospitals. Input into the plans from a population health, or health promotion, position, was lessened. We concluded from our analysis that the plans remained a missed opportunity to link health to the planning of the city. Health, despite being considered, remained far from being institutionalised as a core policy objective for infrastructure planning and delivery.

Our comparative analysis of strategic plans in Sydney and NSW showed how the word 'health' appeared to have hit the policy agenda in both plans. This 'health' framing tended to reflect the visualisation of a 'liveable' competitive global economy with world class healthcare facilities. However, at a deeper level, we showed the structural problems facing a healthy planning agenda. Indeed, ideas like liveability paper over these structural cracks (McGreevy et al., 2019, 2020; Pill, 2021). The most significant themes in the plans associated with health were visions for compact, mixed use, walkable and transit-oriented development, subsumed under 'liveability'. But articulating strategies to improve liveability were largely spatially confined to urban areas targeted for residential infill and redevelopment. This over emphasised infrastructure investment to city centres, leaving car dependent and generally lower income, outer metropolitan areas potentially untouched. In addition, the plans emphasised road infrastructure projects as fundamental to urban development. Roads as the only infrastructure option is a hidden contradiction that conflicts with liveability, walkability and transit-oriented development. Ultimately, we concluded that policy conflicts and contradictions meant the policies were unlikely to deliver more healthy and equitable cities without further consideration of some of the structural issues likely to undermine healthy and equitable urban development.

ENVIRONMENTAL ASSESSMENTS OF MEGA INFRASTRUCTURE PROJECTS: A GOVERNANCE FAILURE

Environmental Assessments (EAs) are planning processes established, under legislation (NSW Legislation, 2019), to be the main point at which the public can access and influence decisions about very large infrastructure projects before they are delivered. As such, EAs are the point in the infrastructure lifecycle where planning meets implementation and, perhaps more importantly, communities are given the opportunity to comment on the proposed piece of infrastructure. I use this section to explain, in the light of theory, how this laudable goal was undermined when the planning system set out to approve and deliver these projects for essentially economic growth reasons rather than balance in the public interest. Crucially, this was point of the research where a public engagement/empowerment angle to governance became most visible.

The cases occurred within very different contexts. One set of cases focussed on transport infrastructure projects (2 motorways and a light rail) in highly urbanised Sydney with a comparison motorway project in South Australia. The other set focussed on coal mining projects in the Hunter Valley, a few hours north of Sydney and characterised by a highly populated region with multiple industries competing for space.

For our initial transport mega-project EA research (Harris et al., 2018), I borrowed heavily from a paper about EA practice and theory that revolved around Habermas's 'theory of communicative action' (Elling, 2009). That theorising helped me to differentiate the roles of stakeholders, the system or lifeworld that they inhabit, and flowing from this the substantive goals they see the EA achieving. Positioning values at the centre of practice was particularly interesting to me at the time and was a precursor to the concept of 'hegemonies' that I introduce next chapter.

Elling's use of Habermas'[1] theory helped us critique the tendency in EA circles for EA practice to be considered a rational and objective policy enterprise that positions facts into policymaking. With much chagrin, I recall how a reviewer of one submitted version of the paper to a planning journal rejected the paper with the simple message that 'EIA is an objective assessment of the impacts of a project' and thus our analysis was moot. Rather, in governance terms, the paper showed how the values of stakeholders involved in EA predetermined their engagement with the EA.

Essentially, we found that different stakeholder actors—developers (proponents), administrators, the public, consultants—used EA as a 'means to an end' to achieve specific system goals (Harris et al., 2018). Economic growth and efficiency were the value proponents most adhered to. Administrators aimed to balance least harm with maximum, often economic, benefits. Conversely, the public aimed to reach an understanding about the impact of the project through the EA, questioning both the objectives of the project and the EA as a means to assess this. Beyond local communities, 'the public' also included the wider community, often characterised (in the EA impact statements) as largely benefiting from the projects in economic terms. We also identified the role and positioning of consultants in the EA. Those coordinating the EA acted on behalf of the proponent to progress the project efficiently through the approvals process while coordinating an assessment of the project to minimise its negative impact. The other type of consultant was the technical specialist. Their goal was to deliver the best technical assessment possible, including engaging with the community about that assessment, within the parameters they were given.

The role of different types of government administrators as *either* regulators, advisors or even proponents also came up. The Department of Planning led by the Planning Minister were core administrators. The Department would weigh up, against a range of other impacts, the evidence and issue final conditions of approval for the project to proceed. The Health Department were involved as administrators but did not have nor wanted regulatory authority to approve projects. They felt that their advisory role allowed the health input to be focussed on developing an

---

[1] For an excellent overview of why Habermas never managed to be critical enough about power (and structures) see Flyvbjerg (2001).

objective assessment of whether the risks to health through changes to the environment were adequately assessed within the EA.

EA governance was clearly a mix of public and private practice. The government bureaucracy regulates and reviews the EA process paid for by proponents and undertaken by private consultants. But this arrangement locked out communities from being able to engage with the EA as a meaningful process to influence policy. Communities, it was repeatedly made clear, are under-resourced and disempowered as stakeholders in the EAs. The EAs themselves had become a technocratic area of practice that predetermined not only the issues that could be included, but also who was included in the process.

An administrator's take on coal mining EAs for instance was instructive here:

> I think there needs to be a lot more engagement through the development of EAs and so on, between the community and so on... talking to people a lot more, and actually trying to feed the things they say and value into the weighing up in a more sophisticated way, is fundamental to us doing a better job. I don't think we're going to make all people happy, all of the time. But certainly we are spending a lot of time and effort actually trying to improve the way we deal with the community at every step of our process. (State Planning Administrator)

Two separately undertaken pieces of research into the governance behind WestConnex, undertaken by planners and geographers (Haughton & McManus, 2019; Searle & Legacy, 2021), support and deepen our findings. Both studies found the Environmental Impact Statements (the public document produced from an EA) to be focussed on specific issues of interest to a very narrow band of pro-development stakeholders. Both studies found the EISs occurred too late to do anything but be a final tick of approval for a predetermined project. At a deeper, normative level, informed by theory, both papers argue that that conflict ought to be an inevitable feature of diverse democratic societies. The result of this inevitable conflict is a need, in policymaking, to acknowledge and engage with differing views. The term for this engagement in Planning circles is called 'agonism'. The term is not as clear, in my view, as it could be (agony does not encourage a positive image of debate). Agonism is however used by Planning researchers to explain how differences in voices and views are kept in the foreground rather than 'managed out' by technocratic processes like EAs.

What this body of separate studies (including ours) revealed was how WestConnex was an example of how Planning practices, in neoliberal 'growth/competition' systems, through technocratic processes, overemphasise the positions of private investors and underemphasise community concerns. More recent literature by planning academics explains that this 'post-political', technically driven, approach to planning is the way that policy is made in Sydney (Greiss & Piracha, 2021). Post-political Planning is, it can be concluded, the fundamental 'path dependency' that a public health, health equity, or place based approach must face and challenge. I return to this core finding in the next section on the Western Sydney City Deal.

At the same time, collectively, these studies support the proposition developed in the previous chapter that governance and goals are intertwined. Further, the research shows that power, detailed in the next chapter, is the core mechanism that brings together goals and governance as 'hegemonies'. Haughton and McManus, in their paper, showed how planning processes like EAs are used by governments to 'control the narrative' behind projects such that public debate is stymied unless strongly supportive of the project. Similarly, Searle and Legacy focussed in on how the 'Public interest' becomes sidelined by the narrative being put forward by those in power who use planning processes to frame the discourse surrounding a particular development. Searl and Legacy, like us (Robertson et al., 2021) showed how WestConnex is an example of the public interest in a particular context being 'conditioned on the interplay of structures of power and knowledge' (see also Flyvbjerg, 1998; Flyvbjerg et al., 2003). Our research showed broad public health concerns with the social determinants of health, raised in response to EISs and then a legislative inquiry into the failures of planning for WestConnex, were sidelined in the EAs. Attempts by less powerful actors who do not control the narrative are constrained by restricted planning processes that perpetuate, rather than question, the status quo that suits the interests of the powerful (Haugaard, 2003; Lukes, 2005).

We found the governance of EAs manifestly failed to provide a transparent mechanism for foregrounding disagreements. Indeed, community concerns were largely dismissed by the technocrats in charge of the EAs as being motivated by 'Not in My Backyard' (NIMBY) interests. Or worse. For instance, one participant explained community concerns away as primarily motivated by loss of the prices of people's homes. As if losing or devaluing one's home is not a legitimate concern in and of itself. The result, rather than an opportunity for public input (Cashmore & Kornov, 2013), is subversion of democratic input into the planning process (Swyngedouw, 2009).

The timing of the EA is also problematic given EAs intended community engagement credentials. EAs occur very late in the decision-making process, almost at the end of the project appraisal process, when communities are directly faced with actual projects being constructed. That input is only meaningfully sought at this late-EA stage plays into the perception of EA as occurring for appearances sake only. The late timing also narrows the various options available to the public to understand and engage with. For instance, WestConnex was presented for community input as a fabulous project that was only ever going to be a massive road within very strict geographical boundaries. Notably, participants in the infrastructure and health research, the aim of which was understanding how infrastructure is planned and delivered, uniformly dismissed EA as biased against meaningful policy input (Harris, Riley et al., 2020).

In terms of governance, health input was only invited if it was able to show a project had positive net impacts. What was never in question was whether the project was a good idea for population health in the first case. Why?

We found that the Planning legislation (NSW Legislation, 2019) discourse structures out the possibility of anyone but a select few to put forward reasonable alternatives to the initial concept of the piece of infrastructure. There is no reference in the legislation to developing a full business case, including various options for other types of infrastructure that might be viable alternatives (or not) to the particular project being put forward. These options or alternatives would necessarily need to take into account broad, population wide impacts on health, wellbeing, equity and the climate. But the legislation precludes such processes from being required. Internationally, these limitations of the EA process are well understood. In jurisdictions like the European Union, for instance, expressly to counter the constraints of project by project assessments, options-based assessment processes called Strategic Environmental Assessment (SEA) have been put into place. SEA is not a panacea for public health by any stretch, but it is a better procedural option for population health issues than EA as currently practiced under legislation in Australia. However, I was told by one senior ex-bureaucrat that when the idea for

SEA was put forward to the NSW Department of Planning over a decade ago it was rejected as being yet another hurdle to development.

Despite the land use planning legislation, the NSW Government has recently produced procurement guidelines that clearly lay out the need to understand and assess risks and benefits—health is not mentioned—of particular infrastructure options before isolating and proceeding with one or another (NSW Government, 2021). Reforms towards new way of managing public sector investment came about around the same time I was doing this research. Remarkably as of 2021, the NSW Government admits the need for these reforms to replace an 'outdated and prescriptive policy framework, underpinned by the oldest financial management in Australia' (Treasury, 2021). In contrast, the Federal Government developed guidance for transport planning that exhort infrastructure planning to work across the very long and detailed development of strategic options and then business cases (Commonwealth of Australia, 2016). But in NSW, especially for state significant infrastructure, we showed this type of best practice does not occur. At best, we showed how a small group of decision-makers will put forward various options for different road routes, rather than options for roads vs other types of infrastructure. By the time, the EA process comes around this clearly risks approving what could be the wrong decision for the problem at hand (Flyvbjerg et al., 2003).

Health input, we found, would often be better spent supporting the critical role of planners at earlier strategic points of engagement in the fundamental options for a project. In our original analysis, we showed how one community submission to the EA of WestConnex raised the idea that the health input should have been done on earlier options rather than the already assumed transport modelling for the final project (Harris et al., 2016). This same critique subsequently arose again as a recommendation for reforming planning around mega-projects in response to the Parliamentary inquiry into WestConnex mentioned above.[2] In both instances the Government responses publicly asserted that EA is best practice planning which sits alongside the development of options and business cases. From a governance perspective that response is laughably disingenuous. The reality we showed in our case studies was that the public was never presented with a transparent opportunity for early input into whether

---

[2] https://www.parliament.nsw.gov.au/committees/inquiries/Pages/inquiry-details. aspx?pk=2497#tab-reportsandgovernmentresponses.

public spending on either motorways or coal mines was the best use of public money.

During the coal mining case study (Harris et al., 2021), I came upon the explanatory power of Bourdieu's[3] concept of discursive symbols as narratives that control social systems and planning practices (see Bennett, 2000). Ideas and discourses became, just as Bourdieu suggested, symbols of meaning bearing traces of wider social structures. Capital, for Bourdieu, denotes any institutionalised resource, material or symbolic, capable of conferring access to positions of authority (Neveu, 2018). Discourse symbols like economic capital both express and reproduce those structures, while serving the interests of some groups over others. The state, according to Bourdieu, comprises a range of actors that maintain symbolic power or work to undermine it. Economic capital, I began to see, became the symbol of capital all actors involved with the NSW Planning system seek to enable or disrupt.

As symbols, concerns with public health struggled to either connect with or counter the dominant discursive economic growth narrative. Transport projects were, we showed, conceived, planned and executed based on their 'necessary' functioning as engines of economic capital for the state. Coalmining was similarly positioned, politically, as essential for the economic growth of the state. Similarly strategic planning was essentially an exercise in setting the road map for delivering infrastructure for economic growth, subject to later Environmental Assessment informed approvals. And so the system unfurls.

Following Bourdieu, the economic capital symbol predetermined the governance of the planning process, including EA. This predetermination however weakened the institutional role of 'Planning' to facilitate broader governance input and wide consultation with the public about whether decisions are in their interest or not.

The problem of under-loading the original options behind an infrastructure project was not limited to Transport projects. Coal mining, for instance, was explained as follows:

[3] It is noteworthy that I initially found this line of theory in paper about power within coastal planning in Norway Bennett, R. G. (2000). Coastal planning on the Atlantic fringe, north Norway: The power game. *Ocean & Coastal Management, 43*(10–11), 879–904.

the way the system is set up is very much about mining is a state significant development and so therefore decisions about it are made in Sydney, basically, and the lack of local control and input is part of the social impact of mining...there seems to me to be a fear from government of public input in consultation and I think they think that everybody wants no mining at all and we hate the whole thing or whatever. And so they set up a system so that basically, you didn't have to deal with the fact that the public or the farmers or whoever it was didn't really want it to happen....its just a bunch of Sydney based people who aren't really part of the community making the decision. (NGO representative)

Western Sydney City Deal: New Ideas Hobbled by Old Institutional Interests

The Western Sydney City Deal (WSCD) was developed by the three levels of the Australian government to guide the delivery of infrastructure, particularly the investment in the new Airport in the West of Sydney. The WSCD is a long term commitment (to 2038) and involves multiple billions of dollars of investment. The airport alone is a $5.3 Billion government investment. The opportunity the WSCD presented, which was a long time coming, was seized by the new kid on the block, the Greater Sydney Commission (GSC) to 'deliver' their district plan [for Western Sydney] and give them power and influence over decision-making. At the same time, the plan articulated the fundamental parameters of the WSCD around which governance frameworks were set and activities delivered. We focussed on the discourse in publicly available implementation plans and reports for the WSCD, and interviews with stakeholders involved in the planning (Harris et al, 2022).

This case was the point in the research program where I really delved deeply into the Urban Studies/Urban Politics literature. An important footnote to the analysis is that participants, when interviewed, explained their work on the WSCD as innovative and novel. Several participants proposed how those responsible felt as if they were feeling their way through the process because it was so complex and new. In the light of theory, however, the strategies employed to plan and deliver the WSCD are not novel. Those tasked with the plan were no doubt busy navigating the right language and stakeholders to do something innovative and important for their work and the people of Western Sydney. They were, and are, trying to change political path dependencies with 'new' ways of working—especially the idea of place-based approaches. But at a deeper, political level, the WSCD conforms (even defaulted) to many of the governance strategies to develop a city region that have been documented and critiqued in the past 10–30 years in the literature. One recent Australian critique of the WSCD has complained that rather than being a new policy approach to cities it has defaulted to being 'old wine in new bottles' (Hu, 2019). For instance, struggles to insert place-based approaches into urban policy in Australia, including Sydney, have been documented as far back as 2004 (Fincher et al., 2016; Gillen, 2004; Rushton, 2014). These struggles form the backdrop to the governance analysis presented here.

Participants explained the WSCD as essentially a new form of urban governance. There was the sense that the governance, for them, was the most innovative aspect of the WSCD. In the Australian context, the WSCD brought the three layers of Australia's federated government system together for the first time in the development of a city region. The historical challenges facing this tri-governmental approach were (and are) enormous. The work of the GSC in particular to create a governance framework is an instance of what Healey (2006) emphasises as the ultimate power game new institutions when grappling with established path dependencies.

The institutionalised challenges to that 'new' governance framework were explained as follows at each level.

The governance challenges that the Australian federation brings have been previously described as formidable for public policy (Painter, 2001). Federalism was a particular challenge for urban policy, participants suggested, because of an historical aversion within the Federal government to invest in cities, particularly via local government. Capturing Federal investment attention via the airport was fundamental to the WSCD.

At the state government level, the GSC was a new planning institution placed initially inside the NSW Government with a very new ethos in their approach to city planning, which was described as place-based and is detailed below. The GSC was viewed by all participants as (with the WSCD as a specific example) being established as a 'disruptor' to the history in Sydney for top down, centralised and sector specific, or siloed, government planning.

All participants explained how the GSC's approach to urban politics was at odds with the approach of the Department of Planning, under whom the GSC originally sat. In mid-2018 the GSC shifted to the Premier's Department (DPC). That shift was explained by all participants as a 'major win' because this provided the remit to work across government. The reality, however, was that a centralised approach remained part of the culture of the Premier's Department, which threatened the governance behind the WSCD and the aspirations of moving to a place-based approach.

For Local Government, an historically uncooperative or competitive relationship between councils was the reason why the coordination of the eight local councils under the WSCD was explained by most participants as a major governance success. That collaboration was explained—see also Pierre and Peters (2012)—as coming about through strategic vision and persistence of certain high level, long serving and council staff. These individuals initiated the idea of the WSCD as an opportunity for councils to collaborate and leverage resources for the region, and the 38 commitments as accountability mechanisms. Collaboration on the WSCD was largely viewed as being supported because councils recognised how, through co-operation, they could achieve more compared to their previous siloed ways of working. Several participants from local government noted, however, that not all councils in the region had signed up; a situation described as an 'impediment' to the equity aspirations behind the WSCD. Notably the omission of that large council also negatively influenced the engagement of the local health district that covered that council area, who engaged less proactively because of this omission.

All participants explained how the GSC took responsibility for setting up this governance framework (including a 'Delivery Office', resourced by State government where the three levels of government work together to implement the WSCD). Essentially, the governance approach the WSCD took (Morrison & Van Den Nouwelant, 2020) conforms to the emphasis in the literature on government at the centre with additional public–private partnerships where infrastructure was to be financed and delivered (Healey et al., 2002a, b). The WSCD's approach to governance thus resonates with what Jessop, in the public administration literature, explains as 'heterarchies' (Jessop, 1998). These, essentially, are governance networks across actor types to share resources to achieve 'mutually beneficial' goals. Heterarchies, Jessop explains, are based on long term goals, short-term objectives and harnessing the capacity of those involved for different activities and responsibilities across the public sector (government); thereby establishing the groundwork for public and private investment.

Governance, essentially, requires resources to achieve an outcome deemed mutually beneficial. That necessarily involves struggles to disrupt previous power dynamics and path dependencies (Jessop, 1998; Stoker, 1998). Under such complex, power laden, conditions the literature highlights two crucial mechanisms that help describe the governance in the WSCD. First is negotiating commitments for change among existing power dynamics (Jessop, 1998). The ability of the GSC, for instance, to negotiate across stakeholders was explained by most participants as 'soft governance'. Soft governance was in fact described as the most important skill the GSC brought to the WSCD. Second is creating legitimacy through a mandate that gives institutional power to achieve change (Stoker, 1998). Participants explained how the GSC-created legitimation for their work on the WSCD primarily through gaining the support of the Premier (and to a lesser extent Cabinet) and being given formal responsibility for achieving the WSCD.

All participants identified individual entrepreneurial leaders as critical to negotiating the WSCD in the face of the siloed workings of government. In this way, individual agency was, up to a point, able to overcome institutionalised path dependencies (Lowndes, 2009). The long term success of governance, however, requires establishing institutional capacity (Healey et al., 2002b). Interpersonal skill can only go so far and the literature is clear that governance 'success' also requires establishing ongoing mechanisms for inter-agency checks and balances to manage the ever present risks of failure (Jessop, 1998; Stoker, 1998). The task is to move beyond the influence of a few already powerful elites (Healey et al., 2002a, b; Swyngedouw, 2005) by mixing 'hierarchical' with 'network governance' (Rode, 2019) to establish heterarchies (Morrison & Van Den Nouwelant, 2020). In 2018,[4] it was not at all clear whether institutional flexibility had been established. Most crucially, limited engagement with communities

---

[4] Writing in 2021, I have become actively involved in the Western Sydney Health Alliance. My experience gives a positive perspective on governance. The Western Parklands City—which has taken over as the focus from WSCD—is, as heterarchy theory suggests, based on varied objectives and a focus on different layers of stakeholders. Indeed, those involved in the governance are themselves bemused by, as well as accepting of, its complexity. They also, from my recent experience with trying to insert health and equity into these layers, accept that power is fundamental to achieving change. The approach remains a government led, statist and focus. Communities, notably, remain at a distance.

absence undermined attempts at addressing health and equity (Corburn, 2017). I come back to that problem, essentially an issue of power, in the next chapter.

'Place-based planning' might have been a useful and important phrase for participants, but in practice in the WSCD was limited. The actual application of 'Place-Based planning', at the time of the research, conformed to a largely top-down government driven process to coordinate infrastructure investments for agglomeration (Scott & Storper, 2015). Notably, the community, social services and social housing sectors were excluded from the WSCD. Importantly, the approach differed entirely from bottom-up concepts of 'place-based policy', which engages community members and social services at a local level in activities to improve health or social capital (Bradford, 2005). Indeed, when pressed about community engagement most participants explained that a bottom-up approach of active community engagement had not been undertaken at the time of interviewing. Thus, despite the plan mentioning '*putting people first*' in rhetoric this did not occur in practice. The risks of top-down approaches to governance are made clear in the literature in that such processes tend to shore up existing power relations, limiting transparency and democratic accountability (Healey et al., 2002a, b; McCann, 2017; Swyngedouw, 2005).

As an idea, participants suggested that placemaking in the WSCD challenged existing path dependencies within urban policymaking. First, infrastructure planning tended to default to the financial cost and economic benefits of particular infrastructure project investments rather than being driven by concerns for its impacts on places and people. Second, 'place' challenged traditional siloed, top down, centralised approaches to governance. Third, place-making committed the government to bottom up rather than top down resourcing. Each challenge notably corresponds to the identified governance barriers to place-making in the literature (PPS, 2016): i.e. that planning is traditionally driven by top down bureaucratic processes focussed on projects designed within disciplinary siloes, and with no meaningful community engagement.

In our original paper (Harris et al, 2022) we demonstrated how the goals and values behind the governance of the WSCD clearly conformed to the 'Pro-growth' dimensions of Pierre's (1999, 2011) framework (Chapter 8, Table 8.1). We also showed how equity aligned with the 'welfarism' dynamics of that framework and thus was misaligned with the governance and power behind the WSCD. We concluded, however, that this false dichotomy between economic and market driven vs equity and welfarism is one that puts the WSCD at great risk from achieving its goals of making infrastructure work for Western Sydney. Put simply, the discourse in the WSCD planning documents avoided any type of risk, such as inequity, because of a predeliction for encouraging global economic investment. The interviews were more circumspect about equity but also tended to default to a rosy picture about the investment credentials of WSCD. Interviewees felt that investment would automatically impact positively on the historical infrastructural and economic inequities faced by the region.

Absences also matter in policy. Most of the urban policy literature is clear that market failure associated with speculative capital accumulation is the greatest risk to governance, with social inequity the major consequence (Harvey, 2001; Jessop, 1998). It is noticeable then that there were several clear market-based risks in the WSCD not articulated in the plan nor the interviews. One is a downturn in the global economy; another is the strong reliance on a new airport in the face of the need to reduce the use of fossil fuels to mitigate climate change. Perhaps the ultimate governance challenge in the WSCD is ensuring actions to manage these risks are embedded in the delivery of the WSCD.

During the writing of this book, COVID-19 impacted: the global economy took a sharp dive, and the aviation industry ceased functioning, and a series of climate change driven flooding events occurred exacerbated by overdevelopment in Western Sydney. Western Sydney, at the time of writing, was characterised in the media as being Sydney's epicentre of COVID-19. In large part, this occurred because of the 'critical infrastructure' nature of employment and cultural diversity in the region.[5] These risks had not been factored into the design of the 'pro-growth'[6] WSCD in any way.

Complaining that a one in 100-year pandemic was not factored into decisions around the WSCD is on the surface a harsh criticism. However, the goal of economic capital investment-based city competitiveness excluded any reference to risks to public health. The resulting

---

[5] https://www.theguardian.com/australia-news/2021/aug/13/fear-and-loathing-in-western-sydney-how-nsws-covid-response-failed-migrant-communities.

[6] This oversight is again reminiscent of Bent Flyvbjerg's et al., (2003) take down of infrastructure planning and investment across the world as consistently excluding sufficient detail on risks in favour of benefits.

governance, despite the apparent shift to place-based decision-making, shored up existing top-down institutionalised focus on infrastructure for economic growth rather than local placemaking.

Conclusion

In conclusion, this chapter has drilled down into the governance dynamics within the Planning system (in New South Wales) that influenced how health issues were considered and included. Fundamentally, following Bourdieu, I showed how the practice of land use planning and development assessment exists within a wider political narrative emphasising and preferencing economic capital as fundamental for society (Neveu, 2018). Economic capital simultaneously materialised in and created discourses that shaped legislation and practice. This line of reasoning helped explain how infrastructure has come to be positioned in societies like Australia as the core mechanism to manage and progress economic growth. State practices, such as legislation, strategic planning and development assessment were each designed to facilitate infrastructure achieving that economic capital goal. Different aspects of each case showed how health as a policy intersected (or did not) with this core symbol of economic growth.

The long term—10 year—focus of the research helped demonstrate how the planning system is buffeted by competing interests about, ultimately, symbolic capital. At extremes, these positions orient either to economic growth or 'balanced' sustainability. The findings suggested an ongoing battle between these two positions. The positioning of health as a policy issue became caught up in those battles.

That discursive battle over the decade was driven by the core ongoing tension around 'development'. Communities raised concerns and sometimes win in the courts or legislature. Then the government responded by wanting to change the legislation. Then there was a general public outcry on the back of some strategic advocacy work. The government then either backed down or tried to amend the legislation out of sight of the public. One of the interesting tensions that came apparent in the case studies is that the government appears to be operating on the basis of supporting infrastructure for the benefit of society, whereas opposition to infrastructure usually comes about at local levels.

In our original analysis of coal mining environmental assessments, for instance, we provided examples of how communities had 'wins' over industry in the land and environment court (Harris et al., 2021). These judgements effectively turned on evidence provided in environmental assessments which focussed on local amenity and global climate change. However, we also showed how these legal decisions almost immediately triggered the government, overnight in one case, to amend the legislation such that 'economic' concerns held more power than 'environmental' or 'social'.

I also suggested that reform is afoot, especially financing of infrastructure. I suspect that reform has come about in large part due to the dissatisfaction of many within and outside of government with the Planning system and its (mis) use of public funds. Health, broadly defined, however, is not yet part of that reform discussion.

The WSCD has proved to be a case worth watching further from a health and equity perspective. There are currently clear inadequacies appearing in the governance model that conform to a business as usual approach to top down planning from an economic investment perspective (see also Pill, 2021 for a similar analysis of City Deals in general). The shift to place-based (infrastructure) is opening up opportunities for health and equity. But for health issues to be meaningfully considered a better governance approach that accepts input from diverse stakeholders, especially the community, about a diverse set of interests and risks, is required. How Western Sydney land use planning is interfacing with infrastructure has relevance for the global shift towards 'levelling up' disadvantaged regions (Connolly et al., 2021).

As a final point, I can't help but add my normative two cents now, presaging Chapter 11. There is no reason why the involvement of the social services (welfare) sector or civil society in the WSCD would not normally be part of a 'new urban governance' (Kjaer, 2009; Peters, 2019). Engagement with the social services sector and civil society ought to be part of the heterarchical approach to network governance. Such a mixed approach would be inclusive while recognising the need for services as a safety net for the vulnerable, as an employer, and as a connector to the community. The governance behind the planning and delivery of infrastructure in Western Sydney Parklands would benefit enormously from health and equity focussed input.

References

Bennett, R. G. (2000). Coastal planning on the Atlantic fringe, north Norway: The power game. *Ocean & Coastal Management, 43*(10–11), 879–904.

Bradford, N. J. (2005). *Place-based public policy: Towards a new urban and community agenda for Canada.* Canadian Policy Research Networks, Work Network.

Cashmore, M., & Kornov, L. (2013). Changing theory of impact assessment. In A. Bond & R. Howitt (Eds.), *Sustainability appraisal: Pluralism, practice and progress. Natural and Built Environment Series* (pp. 18–33). Routledge.

Commonwealth of Australia. (2016). Australian transport assessment and planning guidelines department of infrastructure and regional development. Department of infrastructure, transport, regional development, communication and the arts. Canberra, Australia.

Connolly, J., Pyper, R., & van der Zwet, A. (2021). Governing 'levelling-up' in the UK: challenges and prospects. *Contemporary Social Science, 16*(5), 1–15.

Corburn, J. (2017). Urban place and health equity: Critical issues and practices. *International Journal of Environmental Research and Public Health, 14*(2), 117.

Elling, B. (2009). Rationality and effectiveness: Does EIA/SEA treat them as synonyms? *Impact Assessment and Project Appraisal, 27*(2), 121–131.

Fincher, R., Pardy, M., & Shaw, K. (2016). Place-making or place-masking? The everyday political economy of "making place." *Planning Theory and Practice, 17*(4), 516–536.

Flyvbjerg, B. (1998). *Rationality and power: Democracy in practice.* University of Chicago Press.

Flyvbjerg, B. (2001). *Making social science matter: Why social inquiry fails and how it can succeed again.* Cambridge University Press.

Flyvbjerg, B., Bruzelius, N., & Rothengatter, W. (2003). *Megaprojects and risk: An anatomy of ambition.* Cambridge University Press.

Gillen, M. (2004). Promoting place: Elevating place-based discourse and new approaches in local governance in New South Wales. *Urban Policy and Research, 22*(2), 207–220.

Greiss, G., & Piracha, A. (2021). Post-political planning in Sydney: A turn in the wrong direction. *Australian Planner, 57*, 1–10.

Harris, P., Riley, E., Sainsbury, P., Kent, J., Baum, F., & Lane, A. (2016). *Assessing environmental impacts of major transport infrastructure projects: Where does human health fit?* University of Sydney.

Harris, P., Kent, J., Sainsbury, P., Riley, E., Sharma, N., & Harris, E. (2020). Healthy urban planning: An institutional policy analysis of strategic planning in Sydney, Australia. *Health Promotion International, 35*(5), 1251.

Harris, P., McManus, P., Sainsbury, P., Viliani, F., & Riley, E. (2021). The institutional dynamics behind limited human health considerations in environmental assessments of coal mining projects in New South Wales, Australia. *Environmental Impact Assessment Review, 86*, 106473.

Harris, P., Riley, E., Dawson, A., Friel, S., & Lawson, K. (2020). "Stop talking around projects and talk about solutions": Positioning health within infrastructure policy to achieve the Sustainable Development Goals. *Health Policy, 124*(6), 591–598.

Harris, P., Riley, E., Sainsbury, P., Kent, J., & Baum, F. (2018). Including health in environmental impact assessments of three mega transport projects in Sydney, Australia: A critical, institutional, analysis. *Environmental Impact Assessment Review, 68*, 109–116.

Harris, P., Fisher, M., Friel, S., Sainsbury, P., Harris, E., De Leeuw, E., & Baum, F. (2022). City deals and health equity in Sydney Australia. *Health & Place, 73*. https://doi.org/10.1016/j.healthplace.2021.102711

Harvey, D. (2001). *Spaces of capital: Towards a critical geography*. Routledge.

Haugaard, M. (2003). Reflections on seven ways of creating power. *European Journal of Social Theory, 6*(1), 87–113.

Haughton, G., & McManus, P. (2019). Participation in postpolitical times. *Journal of the American Planning Association, 85*(3), 321–334.

Healey, P. (2006). Transforming governance: Challenges of institutional adaptation and a new politics of space. *European Planning Studies, 14*(3), 299–320.

Healey, P., Cars, G., Madanipour, A., & De Magalhaes, C. (2002a). Transforming governance, institutionalist analysis and institutional capacity. In *Urban governance, institutional capacity and social milieux* (pp. 20–42). Routledge.

Healey, P., Cars, G., Madanipour, A., & De Magalhães, C. (2002b). Urban governance capacity in complex societies: Challenges of institutional adaptation. In *Urban governance, institutional capacity and social milieux* (pp. 204–225).

Hu, R. (2019). City deals: Old wine in new bottles? In M. Evans, M. Grattan & B. McCaffrie (Eds.), *From Turnbull to Morrison: Understanding the trust divide* (p. 8). Melbourne University Press.

Jessop, B. (1998). The rise of governance and the risks of failure: The case of economic development. *International Social Science Journal, 50*(155), 29–45.

Lowndes, V. (2009). New institutionalism and urban politics. *Theories of Urban Politics, 2*, 91–105.

Lukes, S. (2005). *Power: A radical view*. Palgrave Macmillan.

Kjær, A. M. (2009). Governance and the urban bureaucracy. In J. S. Davies & D. L. Imbroscio (Eds.), *Theories of urban politics* (pp. 137–152). Sage.

McCann, E. (2017). Governing urbanism: Urban governance studies 1.0, 2.0 and beyond. *Urban Studies, 54*(2), 312–326.

McGreevy, M., Harris, P., Delaney-Crowe, T., Fisher, M., Sainsbury, P., Riley, E., & Baum, F. (2020). How well do Australian government urban planning policies respond to the social determinants of health and health equity? *Journal of Land Use Policy, 99,* 105053.

McGreevy, M., Harris, P., Delany-Crowe, T., Fisher, M., Sainsbury, P., & Baum, F. (2019). Can health and health equity be advanced by urban planning strategies designed to advance global competitiveness? Lessons from two Australian case studies. *Social Science & Medicine, 242,* 112594.

Morrison, N., & Van Den Nouwelant, R. (2020). Western Sydney's urban transformation: Examining the governance arrangements driving forward the growth vision. *Journal of Australian Planner, 56*(2), 73–82.

Neveu, E. (2018). Bourdieu's capital (s): Sociologizing an economic concept. In T. Medvetz & J. Sallaz (Eds.), *The Oxford Handbook of Pierre Bourdieu* (pp. 347–374).

NSW Government. (2015). Greater Sydney Commission Act 2015 No 57. NSW Legislation. NSW Government.

NSW Government. (2021). Infrastructure procurement framework. Infrastructure NSW. NSW Government.

NSW Legislation. (2019). Environmental Planning and Assessment Act 1979 No 203. https://www.legislation.nsw.gov.au/#/view/act/1979/203

Painter, M. (2001). Multi-level governance and the emergence of collaborative federal institutions in Australia. *Policy & Politics, 29*(2), 137–150.

Peters, B. G. (2019). *Institutional theory in political science: The new institutionalism.* Edward Elgar Publishing.

Pierre, J. (1999). Models of urban governance: The institutional dimension of urban politics. *Urban Affairs Review, 34*(3), 372–396.

Pierre, J., & Peters, B. G. (2012). Urban governance. In K. Mossberger, S. E. Clarke, & P. John (Eds.), *The Oxford handbook of urban politics.*

Pill, M. (2021). *Governing cities: Politics and policy.* Springer.

PPS. (2016). *Placemaking–what if we built our cities around places?* Project for Public Places.

Robertson, T. J., McCarthy, A., Jegasothy, E., & Harris, P. (2021). Urban transport infrastructure planning and the public interest: A public health perspective. *Public Health Research & Practice, 31*(2).

Rode, P. (2019). Urban planning and transport policy integration: The role of governance hierarchies and networks in London and Berlin. *Journal of Urban Affairs, 41*(1), 39–63.

Rushton, C. (2014). Whose place is it anyway? Representational politics in a place-based health initiative. *Health & Place, 26,* 100–109.

Scott, A. J., & Storper, M. (2015). The nature of cities: The scope and limits of urban theory. *international Journal of Urban and Regional Research, 39*(1), 1–15.

Searle, G., & Legacy, C. (2021). Locating the public interest in mega infrastructure planning: The case of Sydney's WestConnex. *Urban Studies, 58*(4), 826–844.

Stoker, G. (1998). Governance as theory: Five propositions. *International Social Science Journal, 50*(155), 17–28.

Swyngedouw, E. (2005). Governance innovation and the citizen: The Janus face of governance-beyond-the-state. *Urban Studies, 42*(11), 1991–2006.

Swyngedouw, E. (2009). The antinomies of the postpolitical city. In search of a democratic politics of environmental production. *International Journal of Urban and Regional Research, 33*(3), 601–620.

Treasury, N. (2021). *FMT reforms* from https://www.treasury.nsw.gov.au/bud get-financial-management/reform

CHAPTER 10

Power

Throughout the book I have increasingly referred to the back-and-forth struggle for power between rival discourse communities. This chapter uses the lens of power to explain how those struggles influenced the inclusion of health issues in planning policy.

The power focussed literature was especially helpful in explaining the struggles between different 'hegemonies' or discursive communities (Fonseca, 2016; Howarth, 2010). My initial foray into Habermas' theory of communicative action (Harris et al., 2018b) never reached a full critique of how power structures, institutional mandates and the knowledge and actions of policymakers. That was largely because Habermas' theory never really addresses structural power (Flyvbjerg, 2001). 'Hegemonies', rather, explicitly link structure and agency (Carstensen & Schmidt, 2016). Hegemonies are essentially groups that come together as 'discourse coalitions' to contest or progress particular policy issues. 'Hegemony' was originally coined by Gramsci in the 1930's to emphasise intellectual and moral leadership exercised by a group in society. More recently, a hegemony approach (Howarth, 2010) emphasises the practice of coalition building to open up or close opportunity for social and political resistance and change (Carstensen & Schmidt, 2016).

In this chapter, I use these concepts to help explain how power dynamics played out across the cases. I start with legislation, moving

P. Harris, *Illuminating Policy for Health*, Palgrave Studies in Public Health Policy Research, https://doi.org/10.1007/978-3-031-13199-8_10

to strategic plans and then to infrastructure policy, then environmental assessments of major infrastructure projects, and finally the Western Sydney City Deal. Across the analysis I stick to the fundamentals of structure and agency. Structural power provided the institutional backing or blocking for including health in planning. Agency through individuals and groups allowed or excluded health as a policy issue. The idea of health, or health as a discursive construct for policy and policy change, infused across these structural and agentic dimensions (Carstensen & Schmidt, 2016; Schmidt, 2008).

Risking oversimplification, this was the point that the data showed how hegemonies tended to be of two groupings. In one corner were a mix of public and private stakeholders who wanted to see development for primarily economic growth reasons (everything from jobs and growth through to global competition). In the other were a mix of largely community and public interest (some government, especially local government) stakeholders who questioned whether developments or infrastructure should go ahead.

The Absence of Health at the Legislative Level

Across the life of the 2011–2013 reforms, essentially two hegemonies went head-to-head. In one corner was pro-economic, market oriented and largely State focussed.[1] In the other was a 'balanced' position, largely community focussed. Crucial from a power perspective was that the reforms were opened up by the government for broad community input. However, the government rather heavy-handedly refused, despite growing opposition, to change its core belief about the Planning system primarily being a facilitator of economic growth. That position became easily picked on as a 'growth at all costs' mantra that was undemocratic and would ultimately lead to planning being dominated by private sector interests. The winners of the reforms were initially a relatively small community led group that strategically grew on the back of challenging

---

[1] The State conformed to Jessop's (2007; pp. 9–11) conceptualisation of State Power being more than government but a 'distinct ensemble of institutions and organisations whose socially accepted function [created as hegemonies for a particular purpose, in this case market led development] is to define and enforce collectively binding decisions on a given population in the name of their "common interest" or "general will".

the mantra. Ultimately, that group harnessed the power of public opinion and the support of parliamentarians to reject the reforms.

Health had its moment in the sun towards the end of the reforms. The government was searching for positive messaging and thus supported having a new 'Health' focussed objective. That objective was however irrelevant to the fundamental power struggles that were playing out (Harris et al., 2018a). Meaningful structural change towards healthy public policy did not occur.

STRATEGIC PLANNING: CHALLENGING PATH DEPENDENCIES

I've already documented other points when health issues had prominence in the system, especially the two instances of strategic planning—the 2013 metro strategy and subsequent 2018 metropolitan and district plans for Sydney.

Most of the core power dynamics at play with attempting to influence strategic level planning to take on health came down opportunities and struggles for power that new institutional bodies face within broader existing policy institutions (Healey, 2006). The Planning system was—and remains—essentially a policy institution carrying strong path dependencies towards top down hierarchical, sector specific, city planning. However, over time we were able to trace a shift and an opening up in the discourse. One clear shift was towards greater integration across sectors. The other was a nod to new urban governance and 'place-based' decisions.[2] That NSW now operates on a model of integrated land use, infrastructure, and transport plans is an example of overcoming institutional path dependencies to create new ways of working. However, at the time of the research there were clear challenges to developing the necessary regulatory oversight for this type of integrated planning and infrastructure delivery. The Greater Sydney Commission was in

---

[2] Outside the scope of data collection, the past few years saw a concerted push to legislate and deliver 'Place-based' planning. However, despite that effort and thousands of policy man hours to develop a 'Design and Place' policy, the responsible planning minister was replaced and the policy immediately dropped. https://thefifthestate.com.au/business/government/down-the-memory-hole-design-and-place-sepp-documents-pulled-from-government-websites/

many ways introduced as the agency and instrument to make this integrated approach to infrastructure planning take place. But the real power came from the Minister for Planning, with support of (several, over time) Premiers. With the Planning Minister the GSC eventually won the support of the Premier to support their legislated mandate for integrated planning and infrastructure delivery.

A public health policy approach to cities has, we showed, not been able to keep up with these changes and potential opportunities for influence. The real interest in the Planning and government system about health was and remains health and education precincts for the purposes of economic development and global competitiveness. That limited health focus plays into the hands of the health system, who tend towards their institutional 'core business' of planning hospitals and health care rather than population wide prevention. The multi-scaled, relational approach to planning needed to positively influence population health (and health equity) was not part of the health sector's thinking about cities. The relatively few advocates for health beyond hospital precincts tended to emphasis healthy built environments to enhance healthy behaviours like physical activity. Taking on power in terms of shifting the structures driving planning was not well understood or even recognised. Notably addressing power in policy to improve health and equity similarly requires a multi-scaled, relational approach (Friel et al., 2021; Harris et al., 2020).

Finally, and briefly, the community was rarely involved in a meaningful way in these strategic planning documents. There was a nod to involving the community through consultations, but not anywhere near the type of empowering, knowledge sharing that the literature asks for (as explained in the previous chapter). This was very much a state driven enterprise for state focussed outcomes. Once again, this opened up the question about how meaningful the concept of health became in the plans. Indeed, several participants told me that liveability had been used in the later plans as a proxy for health because the community tended to see health as hospitals. Liveability, however, as explained in the previous chapter, is coopted by the powerful as a mechanism for global competition, thereby becoming misnomer for meaningful healthy urban planning.

INFRASTRUCTURE: SYMBOLS OF ECONOMIC POWER

Moving attention to infrastructure helps explain how the lack of power behind public health as a public policy issue played out in decision-making. In the previous chapter I detailed how infrastructure became a discursive symbol for economic growth. Rather than positioning infrastructure for economic purposes as interweaved with social and other forms of capital, infrastructure policy tended to take a narrow view of economic capital. Cost benefit analysis as the main technical process behind infrastructure planning was a good example of that narrow position. Health (and other social impacts like wellbeing) was largely excluded as difficult or too fuzzy cost. There were moves towards engaging with social infrastructure and quality of life as a mechanism to connect different types of infrastructure in the public interest. However, public health was often conflated with those social or quality of life issues rather than being a valued concept in and of itself.

Public health was caught in a power and governance trap. On the one hand there was no meaningful interest or engagement with infrastructure as a determinant of health. Within the health sector hospital financing reigned and fell under the dominant policy discourse of medical and clinical services. This antipathy was mutually reinforced by very few people in infrastructure or urban planning understanding what public health is and what its value for planning and infrastructure delivery is. Infrastructure policymaking, I found, was (and remains) a relatively niche discursive policy community. Public health, with poor framing and lack of institutional mandates and limited interest, was not in a position to challenge the core ideas of that infrastructure hegemony.

ENVIRONMENTAL ASSESSMENTS AND POWER

We found that environmental assessments (EAs) as practiced in NSW were never intended to challenge power. Rather, EAs were a technocratic process to approve projects that occurred so late they had no bearing on whether a project of focus was a good or bad idea.

As it turns out, by the time the EA was undertaken (for the purpose of approving projects), when issues have already been set in the requirements, the fundamental characteristics of the project could not be changed. Negotiation about those fundamentals (weighing up the costs and benefits of roads or public transport alternatives for instance) was not the function of the EA. Conducting the EAs, therefore, necessitated managing the narrowly conceived risks of the project within those fundamental parameters rather than assessing the known pathways linking the project to health.

Structurally, we were able to situate the practice of EA as driven by the legislation. The result was localised, project by project assessments with limited ability to focus at a cumulative or population health level. That legislation predetermined the approval focus of the EA process and the resulting technocratic emphasis on minimising risk, rather than engaging in wider debates about the merit of fundamental decisions for population health. Approvals, we were told, drove EAs purpose and function. This begs the question about the legitimacy of the EA process for stakeholders that might be opposed to projects or to ideas that deviate from those who want a project to go ahead. EA remains a very limited, late, project focussed, procedural point to raise population health concerns about the strategic impact of projects on communities, cities and regions.

Crucially, the decision-making power behind these types of infrastructure project, under legislation, lie with the elected Planning Minister and under [him] with the Department of Planning. The legislation was amended in the 2000's to remove local government as a decision-making authority. Local government can comment on Environmental Assessments or be nominated as an authority to be formally engaged with. The legislation also states that 'state planning policies' have more authority than local environment plans (although in practice, and in case law including those related to coal mines local environmental plans are included in EISs and judgements.[3]

'Health' focussed stakeholders have tended to be caught in the 'expert' technocratic, economic capital hegemony. That limited engagement occurs despite their perception of themselves as providing objective and technical evidence to inform decisions. Bizarrely, this puts those whom the health department intends to protect from the projects, the community, in an opposing, or at least distrustful, position about the merits of that health data. We found many instances where the community felt the health data was subsumed in the modelling assumptions behind the whole project—see also (Flyvbjerg et al., 2003; Morgan, 2012; Richardson, 2005). The main point of public contact in EAs was through public

---

[3] http://www.austlii.edu.au/cgi-bin/viewdoc/au/cases/nsw/NSWLEC/2019/7.html.

meetings where tensions often ran high as the community questioned the technical presentation of data that had already been negotiated. Rather than empowering the community with knowledge (Haugaard, 2003) about the evidence of health impacts of the project, the technical health assessments were accused by the community of being co-opted to the political imperatives behind the projects.

Theories of power triggered particularly useful insights as to why this subjugation of health as an idea for EA occurred. Particularly useful was Haugaard's analysis of power in society (Haugaard, 2003), previously proposed as useful for analysing EA practice (Cashmore et al., 2010). As well as EAs becoming a form of institutionalised 'power over' communities, the idea of health has been caught in what Haugaard calls 'the reification' of knowledge. This reification of knowledge perpetuates issues like health or social, impacts as secondary when compared to environmental issues. The institutional emphasis of the health department on quantifying health risks plays into this reification. However, even quantitative health risk assessment is unable to match the certainty levels of the hard sciences, and so its relevance is questioned. Further, quantitative health risk assessment might be useful in some instances, but we also showed it fundamentally disempowers communities and other stakeholders. This was particularly stark when, as detailed in Chapter 7, we were told the health department explained to communities that they were unable to provide a risk assessment because the population of the communities was too small to generate a significant result.

At the same time different types of knowledge are becoming powerful forces for decisions, but health input into EA has not shifted to accomodate or support that shift. Over the past decade legal challenges, which often include information from an EA, have been used to successfully refuse coal mining projects on the grounds of social amenity and climate change. We showed how the standard consideration of health risks that tend to assess environmental triggers like air and soil are usually characterised in EAs, and resulting legal judgements that use EAs as information source, as supporting the project to go ahead. Both social amenity and climate change based legal decisions are therefore necessitating a broader approach to considering health in EA. Social amenity and climate change, however, challenge the scope of health input and knowledge into EAs to be more accepting of the social determinants of health. Further, social amenity was noted by decision-makers we spoke to as inherently being less certain than other EA impacts and requiring a different approach to assessing impacts. Climate change impacts require new types of knowledge too. Notably running counter to the project by project emphasis driven by an outdated regulatory system, climate impacts are multi-scalar—local to regional to international—and therefore threaten, with good reason, the whole legislative model that EAs are based on. The hegemony of environmental health risk assessment advocates advising the Planning department about health knowledge in EAs were clearly reifying a limited type of knowledge for the communities they are meant to protect.

Power and the Western Sydney City Deal

Economic capital was undoubtedly the central force behind the WSCD—as both a structural and agentic influence. The WSCD deal conforms to a neoliberal, post-Keynesian approach to urban political economy that positions regions as spatial fixes for international capital investment (Brenner, 2019; Harvey, 1989). Just as urban theorists like Brenner and Harvey explain, the main mechanism was using public funds and government driven activity to shore up private investment, with an infrastructure mega-project as the principle (economic) focus. The airport became that economic catalyst for the WSCD. This goal, we showed, oriented the power dynamics of the governance behind the WSCD to one that was about public and private investment, to the exclusion of other stakeholders, issues and risks, particularly the social service sector, civil society and the public (Harris et al., 2022). Overlapping with the governance analysis of the last chapter, structurally, the new entrepreneurial governance approach of the WSCD was incompatible with (or blind to) the need for direct public investment in social goods that need to be in place to service the population (Pierre 1999). This blindness conforms to Pierre's normatively based governance framework, critiqued in Chapter 8 from a normative positions, where 'welfarism' was sidelined in the quest for pro-growth governance. This meant that power behind the WSCD was concentrated into investment and market forces rather than risks from climate change, housing affordability, public health pandemics, and other causes of deep and stark health inequity.

Even the concept of place-making was filtered by several interview through pro-growth city region lens to bring industry on board:

There's a big seminar, real big thing next week which is about the aerotropolis, which is designed to start articulating what investment should look like out there, so that's the defence industry and the housing industry, and so what you're starting to see is, and this is all soft governance, is the relevant people being brought together to start the conversations.

However, others seemed to suggest a reticence to engage fully with industry at the early point in the planning behind the aerotropolis.

Councils are getting proposals left, right and centre. Everyone wants to jump on the bandwagon and make a lot of money quickly. So that's one thing is you do need, government does need to be very blinkered and put aside private enterprise and make, put certain foundational pieces of sound public policy decisions in place first before you start to engage around people who are quite rightly wanting to make a profit. There's nothing immoral or wrong about that. We want them to make a profit, but it has to be done in the right way.

These two quotes are indicative of the need for a mix of hard—structural, regulatory—and soft—agentic, negotiation—power. Both types of power, participants explained, were needed to guide a policy initiative that manages multiple interests around land development and investment. Structurally, the WSCD itself became the opportunity to wield what was explained by participants as 'soft governance'. The whole strategy behind the GSCs management of the WSCD was to manipulate the power dynamics within government to work towards a new form of 'urban governance' that was place—based, and, by extension, more amenable to focussing on health and wellbeing. I put the concept of 'soft power' to the GSC representative who was responsible for the WSCD. The response was that the mechanism for change was soft power, because this allowed a governance arrangement that was flexible rather than static (Healey, 2006; Jessop, 1998) in order to be innovative and responsive to the power held by different stakeholders involved:

The city deal is an example of a soft governance arrangement, you have a look at the best innovation cities, the most inclusive cities, the cities that actually manage the equity through the best...So I'm not interested in the hard governance, I'm not interested in regulation and legislation so much, I'm interested in the soft governance, the arrangements that are fragile because in that fragility comes a need to be vigilant to keep the relationships healthy.

Agentic power is notable in this comment about keeping relationships healthy in a politically fragile environment. This view of agency has similarly proposed in the literature as the principal mechanism to achieve change in the face of structural barriers (Lowndes, 2009) and institutional path dependencies (Healey, 2006; Immergut, 2006):

> The only reason that we have three levels of government cooperation anywhere in Australia is because of the people, I talk about the football team, you need somewhere between 10 and 15 people that actually make these things happen. If you don't have the right ingredients at the federal level, state level and local government level it just doesn't happen.

Despite the power exerted by powerful individuals, the ideas they were pushing largely conformed to the dominant concept of economic capital in the WSCD, and specifically agglomeration. I have already explained how other policy frames and ideas, like disadvantage, and social services that did not fit that perceived economic investment model were not fully engaged in the hegemony driving the WSCD.

Ultimately, the lack of engagement with civil society and the community became the major limitation in the planning for the implementation of the WSCD. There are two potential defences for this position. One was pragmatic, in that those responsible for the WSCD negotiations felt they were setting the framework for later engagement to occur. Second is that in the Australian and especially Sydney context, public engagement is subject to a culture in which government has a greater foothold on life than in 'small government' contexts like the US and in more recent times the UK. Local government in particular sees itself as acting on behalf of the local community. That said, the lack of engagement with the local community about what the WSCD is and what it is trying to achieve was a major blind spot and missed opportunity for local empowerment and engagement. The power focussed urban politics literature is clear that policy initiatives which insufficiently engage with the community up front risk democratic accountability to the communities that they are intended, at least on paper, to benefit (McCann, 2017; Pierre, 2011; Pierre & Peters, 2012; Swyngedouw, 2005).

Rather than being engaging and empowering, the community were locked out of negotiations behind the airport (Haigh et al., 2020). Recent media coverage is replete—for example (Cox, 2021)—with stories of corruption and governance failures surrounding the financing of the land in and around the airport. From a local perspective on urban politics and power, these experiences echo decades of cautions in the literature about infrastructure investment fostering local 'coalitions of property developers and financiers' (Harvey, 1989), and failing to move beyond the influence of a few already powerful elites (Healey et al., 2002; Swyngedouw, 2005). The Minister for Planning recently responded to this negative media by appointing a 'community commissioner for the aerotropolis' to advocate for small landowners in the region (NSW Government, 2021). The Commissioner's 2021 report makes 40 recommendations to ensure the WSCD achieves 'a fair and equitable way forward for small landowners in the Western Sydney Aerotropolis'. The crux of this report is that these 9,100 landowners were locked out of discussions across the first 3 years of the planning behind the aerotropolis. The 40 recommendations revolve around three themes: communication and engagement, responses to impacts, and governance. Essentially the report revolves around sharing power by respecting the life world and experiences of those who are most negatively impacted by the aerotropolis.

CONCLUSION

In conclusion, this chapter has demonstrated how including and considering heath in public policy requires addressing and navigating power. Importantly, the analysis presented supports seminal work by Flyvbjerg (Flyvbjerg, 1998) which demonstrated how power controls knowledge in Planning systems, rather than knowledge controlling power. Across the chapter I showed how each of the cases are examples in power working across systems through structure as well as agency. Meaningfully embracing the concept of health as valid and valuable for planning policy and decisions means taking on structure and agency. Attending to structural change—regulation and procedures—as well as agentic change—negotiation and relationships—at multiple layers of the planning system is essential for healthy public policy. The analysis presented showed how the framing of health was unable to connect meaningfully as a salient policy issue across the hegemonies that lie at the heart of the complexities around planning and developing cities and regions. In the next chapter I drill into this dynamic further, from a normative perspective, and provide some recommendations for progressing healthy public policy.

References

Brenner, N. (2019). *New urban spaces: Urban theory and the scale question.* Oxford University Press.

Carstensen, M. B., & Schmidt, V. A. (2016). Power through, over and in ideas: Conceptualizing ideational power in discursive institutionalism. *Journal of European Public Policy, 23*(3), 318–337.

Cashmore, M., Richardson, T., Hilding-Ryedvik, T., & Emmelin, L. (2010). Evaluating the effectiveness of impact assessment instruments: Theorising the nature and implications of their political constitution. *Environmental Impact Assessment Review, 30*(6), 371–379.

Cox, L. (2021, February 17). 'Development should stop': serious flaws in offsets plan for new western Sydney airport. *The Guardian.*

Flyvbjerg, B. (1998). *Rationality and power: Democracy in practice.* University of Chicago Press.

Flyvbjerg, B. (2001). *Making social science matter: Why social inquiry fails and how it can succeed again.* Cambridge University Press.

Flyvbjerg, B., Bruzelius, N., & Rothengatter, W. (2003). *Megaprojects and risk: An anatomy of ambition.* Cambridge University Press.

Fonseca, M. (2016). *Gramsci's critique of civil society: Towards a new concept of hegemony.* Routledge.

Friel, S., Townsend, B., Fisher, M., Harris, P., Freeman, T., Baum, F. J. (2021). Power and the people's health. *Social Science and Medicine, 282*(August), 114173.

Haigh, F., Fletcher-Lartey, S., Jaques, K., Millen, E., Calalang, C., de Leeuw, E., Mahimbo, A., & Hirono, K. (2020). The health impacts of transformative infrastructure change: Process matters as much as outcomes. *Environmental Impact Assessment Review, 85,* 106437.

Harris, P., Kent, J., Sainsbury, P., Marie-Thow, A., Baum, F., Friel, S., & McCue, P. (2018a). Creating 'healthy built environment' legislation in Australia: A policy analysis. Health Promotion International, *33*(6), 1090–1100.

Harris, P., Riley, E., Sainsbury, P., Kent, J., & Baum, F. (2018b). Including health in environmental impact assessments of three mega transport projects in Sydney, Australia: A critical, institutional, analysis. *Environmental Impact Assessment Review, 68,* 109–116.

Harris, P., Baum, F., Friel, S., Mackean, T., Schram, A., & Townsend, B. (2020). A glossary of theories for understanding power and policy for health equity. *Journal of Epidemiology and Community Health.* JECH-2019-213692.

Harris, P., Fisher, M., Friel, S., Sainsbury, P., Harris, E., De Leeuw, E., & Baum, F. (2022). City deals and health equity in Sydney Australia. *Health & Place, 73.* https://doi.org/10.1016/j.healthplace.2021.102711

Harvey, D. (1989). From managerialism to entrepreneurialism: The transformation in urban governance in late capitalism. *Geografiska Annaler: Series B, Human Geography, 71*(1), 3–17.

Haugaard, M. (2003). Reflections on seven ways of creating power. *European Journal of Social Theory, 6*(1), 87–113.

Healey, P. (2006). *Urban complexity and spatial strategies: Towards a relational planning for our times.* Routledge.

Healey, P., Cars, G., Madanipour, A., & de Magalhães, C. (2002). Urban governance capacity in complex societies: challenges of institutional adaptation. In G. Cars, P. Healey, A., Madanipour, & C. De Magalhães (Eds.), *Urban governance, institutional capacity and social milieux* (pp. 204–225).

Howarth, D. (2010). Power, discourse, and policy: Articulating a hegemony approach to critical policy studies. *Critical Policy Studies, 3*(3–4), 309–335.

Immergut, E., M. (2006). Historical-institutionalism in political science and the problem of change. *Understanding Change,* 237–259. Springer.

Jessop, B. (1998). The rise of governance and the risks of failure: The case of economic development. *International Social Science Journal, 50*(155), 29–45.

Lowndes, V. (2009). New institutionalism and urban politics. In Jonathon Davies and David Imbruscio (Eds.), *Theories of urban politics,* 91–105.

McCann, E. (2017). Governing urbanism: Urban governance studies 1.0, 2.0 and beyond. *Urban Studies, 54*(2), 312–326.

Morgan, R. K. (2012). Environmental impact assessment: The state of the art. *Impact Assessment and Project Appraisal, 30*(1), 5–14.

NSW Government. (2021). New community commissioner for aerotropolis: Ministerial media release: NSW Department of Planning and Environment. NSW Government.

Pierre, J. (1999). Models of urban governance: The institutional dimension of urban politics. *Journal of Urban Affairs Review, 34*(3), 372–396.

Pierre, J. (2011). *The politics of urban governance.* Palgrave Macmillan.

Pierre, J., & Peters, B. G. (2012). Urban governance. *The Oxford Handbook of Urban Politics.*

Richardson, T. (2005). Environmental assessment and planning theory: Four short stories about power, multiple rationality, and ethics. *Environmental Impact Assessment Review, 25*(4), 341–365.

Schmidt, V. A. (2008). Discursive institutionalism: The explanatory power of ideas and discourse. *Annual Review of Political Science, 11,* 303–326.

Swyngedouw, E. (2005). Governance innovation and the citizen: The Janus face of governance-beyond-the-state. *Urban Studies, 42*(11), 1991–2006.

CHAPTER 11

Normative Critique About Healthy Planning

This chapter completes the research by taking a normative, or what should happen, position.

Critical realists have long been interested in normative positions. Their interest turns on the acceptance that social science 'must be critical of the practices it studies…must have a standpoint from which its critique is made' (Sayer, 2000; p. 173). Sayer nevertheless goes on to explain that normative positions require evidence to support their feasibility and practical adequacy. In my view, linking what one feels should happen is more feasible and practical if supported by evidence about problems and solutions.

Just as policy is value laden, so is scholarship. Chapter 8 revealed clear normative positions among scholars about what 'good' or 'bad' urban policy is. In Chapter 9 and 10 I demonstrated how Pierre's (1999, 2011) paper about urban governance is an example of preferencing pro-growth over other interests such as welfarism. However, healthy public policy advocates have a policy goal of equity (see Chapter 3). For us, pitting economic growth as fundamental for progress flies in the face of evidence about social justice. Note please that we are not alone. For instance, notable urban scholars present similar evidence and arguments (Garcia & Judd, 2012; Pill, 2021). As I pointed out then, and in a recent article about health and political science (de Leeuw et al., 2021), 'unwavering

P. Harris, *Illuminating Policy for Health*, Palgrave Studies in Public Health Policy Research, https://doi.org/10.1007/978-3-031-13199-8_11

support of city region competition driven by market mechanisms is ultimately, and fundamentally, challenged by a social equity critique'. Indeed, it may be that urban scholars like Pierre, brilliant and influential thinkers though they may be, are insufficiently reflective of their own values. Why, for instance, does Pierre (1999) differentiate 'welfarism' from 'growth'? As I noted in Chapter 8, a deeper dive into his paper sees him write that welfare is 'anticapitalistic' and 'needy for private investment but least geared for attracting such investment' (1999, p. 387). However, the reality is that spending on addressing inequity and capital for infrastructural agglomeration need not be diametrically opposed. Indeed, a deeper analysis of the 'growth' agenda suggests successful economies require as much, if not more, of the investment that Pierre so damningly accuses 'welfare' of draining (Pickett & Wilkinson, 2010).

I faced my values head on during the Western Sydney City Deal analysis (Harris et al., 2022). I took a positive but critical position about health equity. During the interviews, the impression all participants gave was one of trying to do the best they could to deliver infrastructure investment (via agglomeration) to lift up the community of Western Sydney in the face of historical under-investment. I remember several interviewees—recalling these people were in powerful positions of influence—raising the WSCD as 'once in a generation' opportunity to rebalance infrastructure investment to favour Western Sydney. But these well meaning folk nevertheless worked in an institutional context that preferenced economic growth and development above all else. In the light of scholarship, their goals, commitments and interests did reflect (see Chapter 8) what McGuirk (2005) has identified as 'resilient elements of a social democratic project ...' in the face of a fundamentally growth-driven neoliberal city region competitive agenda. For me, the analysis challenged whether a public health equity policy agenda was ever going to be able to interact meaningfully with the economic growth focus of initiatives like the WSCD.

During the analysis, I questioned what Healthy Public Policy type engagement means for initiatives that are largely driven by 'strength based' discourse to the exclusion of other issues, positions and risks. Was an equity focus, when narrowly conceived as distribution of disadvantage, too flat rather than nuanced and scaled, too negative rather than positive? At a more fundamental, normative level, I questioned whether the equity agenda is too socialist to be applied to what is clearly a neoliberal endeavour? Or, following Pierre (2009) too 'welfarist' to be seen to add value to the entrepreneurial intentions of the WSCD?

These reflective questions about intersecting values as policy goals were legitimate, it turned out. Indeed, competition between values became a core finding of the analysis. I also realised that these values, in the end, don't need to compete. They do, however, need to be put on the table early in policymaking as issues, risks or benefits to tease out. In the absence of those [health, social, justice, sustainability] equity focussed negotiations, the risks to health are inevitably underplayed in favour of growth at all costs. Eventually, I realised, just as McGuirk (2005) argues, that all the various interests that actors brought to the WSCD take place within a policy context that is driven by market economics, global city competitiveness and mobility of the regional workforce. Through this more nuanced lens, I clearly saw all the WSCD's actors' interests and struggles for influence taking place within the overarching neoliberal city region growth 'pot' (recalling the famous 'garbage can' thesis that permeates through theories of the policy process). That pot/can is the culture of the policy system, reflective as it is of the global neoliberal model of urban competition. There are, however, pockets of opportunities to influence health and equity through the governance and power drivers of that largely growth-driven agenda. But influencing these lies in getting under the skin of the various governance mechanisms that have been put in place to 'deliver' initiatives like the WSCD, now re-branded as the Western Parkland City. Coming full circle and with full disclosure, I have recently been working with the various governance groupings and agencies behind the Western Parkland City to negotiate delivering the 'health' commitment with an equity focus.

For the rest of this chapter, I follow Sayer's suggestion and distil the research findings into lessons for healthy public policy (or at least healthy planning) practice.

LEGISLATE FOR A HEALTH FOCUSSED OBJECTIVE WITH POINTS OF ACTION ACROSS THE SYSTEM

Insert a health focussed objective into legislation governing urban and regional planning. That objective should be worded as necessarily broad (not risks, nor 'within buildings', nor some other narrow conception). An obvious example would borrow from sustainable development (which, by the way, the NSW planning legislation is meant to achieve, as is federal

Australian legislation), with wording like 'the health and wellbeing of present and future generations'. Then, the system then needs to be set up to deliver that objective. As several very senior participants (one a minister) explained when interviewed, legislative objectives are merely the beginning.

A Planning policy focussed on health and wellbeing is required. In NSW, legislation is given effect by State Environmental Planning Policies (SEPP). As of 2021, one was produced about 'design and place'. That policy was driven by the legislative design and place objective of course (yes, this objective came to replace the health objective tabled in the 2013 failed reforms).

Next, strategic and spatial planning instruments ought to be commanded to deliver the health objective with relevant strategies in place. Other instruments, such as 'local environmental plans' for local governments in the NSW context, would then be required to take on the strategic plan's focus as well as that of the health and wellbeing SEPP. Those requirements then feed into local development control plans and into development assessment.

State legislation about development assessment, especially state significant infrastructure, would be amended to deliver the health legislative objective in the business case planning and appraisal for infrastructure projects. Terminology should be expanded to include both 'in the locality' and, crucially, regional and cumulative levels. Yes, developers would be responsible for health and wellbeing impacts that were collectively accumulated and occurred 'outside the fence' of their projects. Perhaps most importantly, the legislation would mandate a full options appraisal, considering public health and wellbeing impacts, risks and benefits, for designated state significant projects or projects considered controversial. That options appraisal would be required to transparently consider infrastructural alternatives (e.g. a mix of transport options, different types of energy, different ways of delivering digital). Further, assessing massive projects in a stage-by-stage manner would only be allowed once a full business case for the whole project had been scrutinised based on a range of options about what the fundamental purpose of that mega-project is, including alternatives and including health and wellbeing considerations.

Local government, civil society and community input about health and wellbeing would be mandated across planning instruments and business cases for state significant infrastructure.

Finally, Planning legislation would link to public health legislation to require input about health and equity impacts broadly defined as social, environmental and commercial determinants of health.

Recommending this type of system reform is not naïve posturing. The recommendations come straight from the evidence I have presented throughout this book. I suppose some readers are concerned that such reforms would unbalance the infrastructure pipeline and put jobs and growth (and political careers) at risk. In response, on the one hand is the irrefutable evidence that the world is quickly hurtling towards a climate-induced death spiral,[1] largely because of the neoliberal market-driven growth focus provided by current legislation and planning systems. That evidence alone is reason enough to make the recommended reforms. On the other hand, it will also be important to evaluate where similar reforms have occurred, or where similar systems have been in place, in terms of how well these function and implications for health and wellbeing (of current and future generations).

LONG-TERM AND STRATEGIC PERSPECTIVE—NAVIGATING INCREMENTALISM IS THE KEY

Across the research, time proved one of the crucial factors, as explained in Chapter 5. Opportunities to bring health ideas, evidence and people to the planning table occurred regularly but incrementally. In addition to major opportunities for 'punctuations' like the 2011–13 reforms, other, more regular but relatively minor opportunities occurred—policy submissions, inquiries, input at a meeting or an advocacy project. Collectively however, what happened when major and minor activity occurred was increased pressure on the status quo to consider and take on what health meant for the system.

Crucially, these opportunities need vigilance on the part of health advocates (Harris & Wise, 2020). Vigilance over the long term is needed to keep momentum, introduce new ideas and then, crucially, ensure the

---

[1] 'Infrastructure and Health: Big Connections for Wellbeing' is the focus of a new Oxford University Press journal (disclaimer, I am editor in chief) https://academic.oup.com/ooih, http://www.austlii.edu.au/cgi-bin/viewdoc/au/cases/nsw/NSW LEC/2019/7.html.

maintenance and relevance of the idea so that it is not replaced. The pressure of the status quo to resist change is enormous, and new ideas struggle for relevance in both the short term and long term.

That vigilance is made much easier when a dedicated resource is in place. Incrementalism requires, just as governance theory and scholarship shows, long-term perspectives, flexibility and resourcing. The Planning system, for instance with the Western Sydney City Deal, has come to realise that a flexible model of governance is fundamental to creating change over time. What is crucial from a health advocacy perspective, as I showed in the last two chapters, is to ensure, with funding commitments and skilled people, a seat at the table with ongoing influence. Only then will health issues be meaningfully considered early on in decision-making and be maintained over the long term.

PICK YOUR BATTLES: BUT PREFERABLY CHOOSE ONE WITH A FUTURE (I.E. SUSTAINABILITY)

Ultimately, the analysis across the research demonstrated the centripetal force of economic growth for the planning system. That market-driven growth goal—more housing, more jobs, more growth!—ruthlessly sucked all other activity towards it. This market-driven agenda was coupled with a path dependency towards new public management and top-down approaches to plan-making and infrastructure investmet and delivery. Both excluded meaningful engagement with health and especially equity as a holistic idea for cities. From a health perspective, the market-driven governance model created two unnecessary bi-products. One was the emphasis on hospital funding and delivery. The other was assessing risk through secondary data to support the approval of major infrastructure projects.

Promoting health can be seen as an appealing goal for urban planning (Barton et al., 2015). Ultimately however, as Steele (2011) articulates, the aim of advocating for change is to transform planning institutions to adopt new ideas and practices as core to their business. As it stands, however, positioning health as a central concept in New South Wales has yet to be institutionalised. Liveability has become a good entry point for health. But without clear articulation of what this means for people's health and how to address existing or future disadvantage, liveability remains a missed opportunity. Over the past decade, despite the yin and yang I have described between of economic growth and balanced sustainability, my sense is that the latter is becoming institutionalised. Politicians might like to think they can dodge evidence. They know they can't dodge public opinion. The reality facing governments in Australia is that the global marketplace for development, and global and local public opinion, has shifted dramatically towards sustainability. At the start of the research, climate change could not be mentioned in the halls of the NSW parliament by either major party. We now, in late 2021, have centre right Liberal environment minister, now treasurer, who has publicly castigated the Federal government for lack of action on climate change.

Our analysis of the legislative reforms reinforced why tying the health argument to the sustainability agenda has deeper roots over the long term. In the short term, democratic accountability, with a goal of balanced sustainability, won out over the pro-business intentions behind the 2011–2013 planning system reforms. With the benefit of longer-term hindsight, the 'balance' position has held strong in the wording of the legislation despite constant threat. At the time of the reforms, there was the sense among health stakeholders that 'we must influence the reforms' with little other strategic intent. That strategy of focussing on the health objective alone was ultimately a mistake despite short-term acceptance of that idea. A longer-term 'health' governance network with the engagement and support of elected officials could have been created/or could be created that taps into an explicit health co-benefit focus to support sustainable, balanced, development.

Framing is a core part of policy. One of the recurrent challenges across the strategic planning cases concerns what type of health issues matter for strategic planning. Participants suggested that healthy planning principles—active living, healthy food, accessible transport—were core to the plans, and therefore, heath was included without explicit mention of the word 'health'. But in my view a 'healthy built environment' framing is insufficient (de Leeuw et al., 2021). Land-use is insufficient. Urban and regional planning has become, as the range of strategic plans we analysed demonstrated, fundamentally about infrastructure for market-driven development. Healthy built environment categories like active living are crucial, but secondary to sustainable development. Of course, taking a relational approach to planning places and spaces (Corburn, 2017; Cresswell, 2014; Healey, 2006) means positively impacting on local built environments. But it also means connecting with the forces behind market-dominated infrastructure. This, I believe, was not and remains not well grasped by healthy planning advocates. Healthy planning needs reflect how cities, their growth and their influence, and the health of their inhabitants, are the result of multi-scalar forces. Healthy planning advocates must understand the political and financial forces behind infrastructural investments, engage across to regulation and policies, and work actively with local communities.

All this attention and framing must be accompanied with a move away from new public management approaches in government decision-making that tend to encourage siloes in both ideas and funding. However, I'm not convinced, based on the analysis presented, that even the shift to new urban governance will shift attention to the wider determinants of urban health. The urban governance literature sees urban politics interacting with health through hospitals or 'service sectors like healthcare' (p. 82) (Pierre & Peters, 2012). This is not because health care is seen as a social good. Rather health care is part of the overall path dependency in planning institutions to foster innovation and a dynamic, creative class workforce that underpins competition between cities (Garcia & Judd, 2012). What is needed, I believe, is a total reframing of health as part of a social equity agenda that balances this 'Planning as economic stimulus' model with other concerns. These concerns are often sidelined in market focussed policymaking, despite their known costs and benefits.

INFRASTRUCTURE AS A DETERMINANT OF HEALTH

Infrastructure has become synonymous in policy circles with societal (usually economic) progress. Healthy public policy advocates have yet to grasp the importance of infrastructure policy and politics. Crucially, infrastructure is influenced by political decisions which are, ultimately, driven by the wants and needs of the public.

For instance, nearly all participants gave the example of how Australian city policy is now driven by knowledge-based rather than manufacturing jobs. Infrastructure needs to respond to this relatively new angle on urban competitiveness. Infrastructure also needs to positively influence health and wellbeing, with equity a crucial consideration. At the time of the research, pre-COVID-19, the core challenge that health and wellbeing posed to infrastructure policy was investment that benefits place-making across the city rather than into flagship mega-projects. Health advocates can and should be involved in and add value to these decisions. The public should be better informed about the positive and negative impacts of those investments.

Quality of life is also an opportunity to include health and equity. There is a tangible shift in the Australian infrastructure sector to engage with quality of life as a core objective.[2] Indeed, in one recent meeting I had with a senior bureaucrat working in infrastructure, I was told that 'what you call public health we call quality of life'. But public health seems to be caught and struggle for relevance; infrastructure policy makers would rather talk about quality of life than public health. This preference may not be fatal, but quality of life without understanding how cities and infrastructure interconnect to create population health outcomes, including who wins and who loses from such decisions, is insufficient. Conversely, public health that does not engage with quality of life as part of the economic focus on infrastructure is similarly insufficient.

In our original infrastructure focussed paper (Harris et al., 2020b), we detail the procedural opportunities for public health in infrastructure policy. Plenty of these, big and small opportunities exist across the infrastructure planning cycle, from strategic level planning to delivery and evaluation of projects. But the main problem is more substantive and institutional. This is a general apathy within the infrastructure sector to the value of public health. There is apathy towards infrastructure as a determinant of health in the health sector. Thus, the siloed nature of policymaking, driven by particular specific sectoral interests, precludes action and meaningful change.

Ultimately, because infrastructure is a sector where there is so much power, money and vested interest, it has almost become unassailable. Decisions and processes became political smoke and mirrors rather than procedures based on transparency and accountability. Public health, in theory and in practice, makes the sector more visible and accountable to the public interest and public scrutiny. Including public health up front in infrastructure planning and business case development is fundamental to opening up better public health engagement with the infrastructure sector. This is not only important for public health, but a potential win–win for the infrastructure sector, which is internally struggling to meaningfully push beyond ongoing politicisation of very large, very expensive, often poorly planned, projects. Environmental assessments

---

[2] https://infrastructuremagazine.com.au/2021/09/03/infrastructure-australia-lau nches-the-2021-australian-infrastructure-plan/.

are a necessary but no longer sufficient entry point for health focussed input.

EAs Need Fundamental Reform

Our analysis of the conditions surrounding the inclusion of health in EA unpacked the dynamics of the planning system with respect to mega-infrastructure projects. The tendency of health focussed research and advocacy is to provide technical evidence to feed into EAs. For some EA focussed practitioners, the institutional forces we unearthed may seem distant from the technical inclusion of health impacts within EA. These forces, we showed, nevertheless exerted a clear influence on that technical practice. The discursive symbol of coal mining or transport mega-projects (especially motorways) as essential for economic capital in society was shown as the fundamental structural level impediment for comprehensive, even meaningful, health input. However, the known impacts of coal mining on health—climate, social amenity—and roads—cars, pollution, physical inactivity, inequity—are largely negative. It follows that when this evidence is included, EAs are likely to challenge the narrative that 'projects are good so they must be built'. That evidence is therefore not included as standard practice in EA. However, without that evidence, the whole system behind EA risks being manipulated to the benefit of industry.

The legislation behind EA itself is at best ambiguous about health and at worst exclusionary. The result is lack of serious consideration about health impacts by industry and in EA practice. This is compounded by health being caught up within a scope of impacts that are classed as less certain than bio-physical impacts on the environment. Discursive ambiguity about health impacts is reinforced by the health department whose advice is that only health risks from changes to air quality are legitimate. But because those assessments were presented on a project-by-project basis, supporting the green light for a project approval, they were distrusted by the communities that the evidence was meant to protect! Moreover, recent legal challenges to coal mining projects, and parliamentary inquiries in to transport projects, are showing that localised health impacts from changes to air quality because of transport or mining activity are insufficient for legal decisions.

Finally, we showed EA practice to be caught between different hegemonies. These hegemonies in EA, we demonstrated, are largely either pro or anti the symbol of infrastructure driving economic growth at all costs.

EA practice is currently oriented towards the former and has become disempowering for the latter. However, at a macro-level, it became clear that the ongoing tension between the two discursive communities reflects broader views about urban and regional development in society and lies at the heart of the whole Land-use Planning system. For health to be a major consideration in EA, the legislation must explicitly include health impacts and be clearer about cumulative impacts across projects or project stages. Health solely positioned as an air quality issue is too narrow. Aligning health within the 'balance' focussed discourse community would align better with the known evidence about the impact of very large, often society shaping, projects.

Our research into EA practice clearly demonstrated the importance of looking beyond a specific technocratic emphasis on the content of EAs to one that engages with the nuances of the approvals system behind massive society shaping projects. The findings have largely been negative, perhaps because an institutional lens to health in EA has not been taken before, thus allowing problematic processes to occur without scrutiny. However, only by looking and deeply understanding the system can points of intervention be developed.

The sufficient inclusion of health in EA requires supportive legislation, guidance on the comprehensive range of links between transport projects and health outcomes, and range of methods beyond risk assessment. Ultimately, the wider process of developing options and business cases is a crucial but missing piece of the infrastructure and health policy puzzle. Ultimately, the culture of government became a major barrier to better consideration of health impacts in EA. The Health Department obsession with air quality as the entry point for health risk assessment was maintained despite the limitations this lens had both for EA practice and for decisions in the land and environment court. The Department of Planning was wilfully ignorant of the value of a broad conception of health for environmental assessments.

Governance Focussed on Health is the Future of Healthy Public Policy

My final point in this chapter concerns governance. In many ways, policy and politics has become all about governance. Who you know is just as crucial as what you know! Similarly, facilitating and engaging in governance networks is perhaps the fundamental for healthy public policy. The range of issues public health overlaps with alone necessitates a strategic and flexible approach to governance for healthy planning. But effective governance also means breaking out of siloes and embracing interests and ideas from other sectors and disciplines, as well as bringing our own ideas and interest to the table. Governance also has a strong institutional flavour and means cementing health and equity goals into policy systems, coupled with building capacity, committing resources, and putting in place actions and strategies to achieve those goals (De Leeuw, 2017).

The Western Sydney City Deal (WSCD) is indicative of the governance task facing healthy public policy advocates. The potential of the WSCD follows years of weak planning and infrastructural investment in Western Sydney. Against that historical backdrop, the WSCD is a promising example of how cities globally can work to break institutional path dependencies. The governance behind the WSCD has, over time, established a multi-level structure to address economic, social and environmental goals. However, without a health and equity lens, governance driven for economic growth above all else challenges engagement to improve social and health equity (see also Pill, 2021). One the one hand, speculative capital accumulation in a volatile global market, especially around air travel in an era of climate change, is the greatest risk to the WSCD and its aspirations to create a health and equitable city region. On the other, a deeper engagement with existing and future vulnerability and disadvantage across the region is essential. Bringing health focussed ideas to the governance table—focussed up, across and down as detailed above—will only enhance the promise of the WSCD for the region.

Conclusion: Ways Forward for the Healthy Planning Agenda

Clearly, the market-oriented pro-growth agenda has power over all governance frameworks and processes in NSW approaches to planning and development assessment. With such a hegemonic power by pro-market forces over the policy discourse, healthy planning advocates are challenged to engage with, create or join existing governance networks. In reality, 'healthy planning coalitions' need to form around either health as a distinct issue for planning (but this is difficult to sustain) or be set up as part of the economic development focussed regimes as a critical check with a social equity perspective. Another, more radical alternative is to create or join 'political' movements that challenge the pro-development hegemony and supporting 'post-political' status quo. These movements, I have shown, do have major influence on the workings of government, particularly when democratic accountability requires policymaking to be opened up to the public.

The analysis presented in this chapter risks being 'bleak' for the health agenda. Here, however, I want to raise a note of optimism as well as propose some suggestions for what is required for change to occur. First, and quite simply, the governance literature is clear that time necessitates change. Given change is inevitable, we need to push it along as well as be ready for it.

Pierre and Peters (2012) articulate several points which help explain the power of governance analysis for healthy planning research, action and advocacy. Urban governance analysis, they argue, is powerful because it articulates the extent to which government is not alone in the process of developing urban and regional policy. Governance necessitates (see also State theory), they argue, a range of other actors beyond government. Opportunities for engagement in governance processes might close or open, depending on the policy objectives being sought. But being involved is crucial. The old adage of politics remains fundamental for healthy public policy; if you are not in the room, you are not part of the conversation.

Pierre and Peters then argue that urban governance theory provides a critical check on the extent to which governance regimes or frameworks deliver on basic democratic requirements like transparency, accountability and popular input. Such ideas, I concur, would open up governance regimes to scrutiny in the public interest. Governance, they conclude, necessitates a focus that balances structure and agency. That observation about structure and agency allows me to come full circle to the analytic spine that has run across this book.

Governance and power in policy ultimately come back to the essential characteristics of institutions—structures, actors and ideas (Harris et al., 2020a; Harris & Wise, 2020). This book, I believe, has provided the analysis to confirm that proposition. Pierre and Peters point out how urban governance in urban studies has allowed analysts to focus on political institutions, political leadership and policy choice in particular contexts. I have similarly shown how the strategic mobilisation of a range of actors in urban politics intertwined with larger goals and objectives that 'structure' political discourse and power dynamics. Pro-market neoliberalism was the clear winner. But if neoliberalism can do that, so can other ideas. The goal of healthy public policy must be institutional transformation towards a healthy, equitable and sustainable future. Power is the challenge. Governance is the mechanism.

References

Barton, H., Thompson, S., Burgess, S., & Grant, M. (2015). *The Routledge handbook of planning for health and well-being: Shaping a sustainable and healthy future.* Routledge.

Corburn, J. (2017). *Equitable and healthy city planning: Towards healthy urban governance in the century of the city* (pp. 31–41). Springer.

Cresswell, T. (2014). *Place: An introduction.* John Wiley & Sons.

De Leeuw, E. (2017). Engagement of sectors other than health in integrated health governance, policy, and action. *Annual Review of Public Health, 38*(1), 329–349.

de Leeuw, E., Harris, P., Kim, J., & Yashadhana, A. (2021, December). A health political science for health promotion. *Global Health Promotion, 28*(4), 17–25.

Garcia, M., & Judd, D. R. (2012). Competitive cities. In K. Mossberger, S. E. Clarke, & P. John (Eds.), *The Oxford handbook of urban politics.*

Harris, P., & Wise, M. (2020). *Healthy public policy.* Oxford University Press.

Harris, P., Baum, F., Friel, S., Mackean, T., Schram, A., & Townsend, B. (2020a). A glossary of theories for understanding power and policy for health equity. *Journal of Epidemiology and Community Health, 74,* 548–552.

Harris, P., Riley, E., Dawson, A., Friel, S., & Lawson, K. (2020b). "Stop talking around projects and talk about solutions": Positioning health within infrastructure policy to achieve the sustainable development goals. *Health Policy, 124*(6), 591–598.

Harris, P., Fisher, M., Friel, S., Sainsbury, P., Harris, E., De Leeuw, E. , & Baum, F. (2022). City deals and health equity in Sydney, Australia. *Health & Place, 73,* 102711.

Healey, P. (2006). Transforming governance: Challenges of institutional adaptation and a new politics of space. *European Planning Studies, 14*(3), 299–320.

McGuirk, P. (2005). Neoliberalist planning? Re-thinking and re-casting Sydney's metropolitan planning. *Geographical Research, 43*(1), 59–70.

Pickett, K., & Wilkinson, R. (2010). *The spirit level: Why equality is better for everyone.* Penguin UK.

Pierre, J. (1999). Models of urban governance: The institutional dimension of urban politics. *Urban Affairs Review, 34*(3), 372–396.

Pierre, J. (2011). *The politics of urban governance.* Palgrave Macmillan.

Pierre, J., & Peters, B. G. (2012). Urban governance. In K. Mossberger, S. E. Clarke, & P. John (Eds.), *The Oxford handbook of urban politics.*

Sayer, A. (2000). *Realism and social science*. Sage.

Steele, W. (2011). Strategy-making for sustainability: An institutional learning approach to transformative planning practice. *Planning Theory & Practice, 12*(2), 205–221.

Postscript

This book has detailed how to analyse, research and progress healthy public policy. Writing the book meant presenting what I hope appears as a coherent whole. I provided distinct sections and chapters. First, I introduced healthy public policy, supported by relevant literature and additional focus on urban health. I then detailed a methodology for healthy public policy analysis and research, supported by literature from critical realism, political science and urban studies. The second part of the book detailed the application of the ideas and methods presented in part 1. The focus was a program of research into urban and regional planning. I first detailed the protocol then presented core empirical findings. I then took a deep dive into relevant theories from a range of disciplines, especially urban politics. In the final section, I used those theories to present a deeper explanation of what happened and what can be done to create a 'healthy' Planning system.

That structure belies the much more unwieldy, iterative process I went through. The methodology allowed that. In fact, my main observation for others planning similar programs is to take an iterative approach. Iteration is necessary when the search for causal explanations is neither uniform nor reductive. Following the methodology presented in Chapter 4, I iterated between collecting data, working through theories searching for explanations, applying those theories, and critically reinterpreting the data considering that knowledge. The result was deep presentation not only of the urban and regional planning system under scrutiny, but also the supporting theoretical knowledge. This was done systematically so that readers can track back my findings both to theory and to the empirical evidence.

The methodology I have used has a long history in the social science. Far fewer attempts have been made to apply the approach offered in this book to the problem of public policy for health, which is the focus of the series this book belongs too. I don't feel the need to repeat lessons and findings here. The book itself has presented and then re-presented those insights in sufficient detail throughout, I think. Suffice to say in conclusion that the methodology works for the problem of illuminating healthy public policy. For inquiry that is non-reductive, requires a relational view of causation and accepts complexity, I hope I have provided a road map to others to use. At the same time, I have navigated how to apply knowledge from a range of sectors to the problem of healthy public policy generally, and healthy urban and regional planning in particular. I hope the eclectic mix of methods and findings appealed to the broad readership this series is written for.

Finally, the core ideas I have presented can be applied to a range of current problems facing the modern world. Generating evidence with a critical lens is a necessary precursor for any society's progress towards being better, more equitable, healthy and sustainable. This book has revelled in the challenge of illuminating policy, critically and systematically, to better understand and explain what is necessary for positive change and progress towards a better, more equitable, healthier, future. I hope others can use the methodology for their research, as well as some of the theories where relevant for their work. Onward!

References

Acheson, D. (1990). Edwin Chadwick and the world we live in. *The Lancet,* *336*(8729), 1482–1485.

Arcaya, M. C., Tucker-Seeley, R. D., Kim, R., Schnake-Mahl, A., So, M., & Subramanian, S. (2016). Research on neighborhood effects on health in the United States: A systematic review of study characteristics. *Social Science & Medicine, 168*, 16–29.

Archer, M. S. (1995). *Realist social theory: The morphogenetic approach.* Cambridge University Press.

Arts, B., & Van Tatenhove, J. (2004). Policy and power: A conceptual framework between the 'old'and 'new'policy idioms. *Policy Sciences, 37*(3–4), 339–356.

Arundel, J., & Lowe, M. H. P. (2017). Creating liveable cities in Australia Mapping urban policy implementation and evidence-based national liveability indicators. Centre for Urban Research, RMIT

Atkinson, A. B. (2015). *Inequality.* Harvard University Press.

Badcock, B. (2014). *Making sense of cities: A geographical survey.* Routledge.

Baert, P. (2005). *Philosophy of the social sciences: Towards pragmatism.* Polity.

Bambra, C. (2016). *Health divides: Where you live can kill you.* Policy Press.

Bambra, C., Fox, D., & Scott-Samuel, A. (2005). Towards a politics of health. *Health Promotion International, 20*(2), 187–193.

Bambra, C., Lynch, J., & Smith, K. E. (2021). *The unequal pandemic: COVID-19 and health inequalities.* Policy Press.

Barton, H., Thompson, S., Burgess, S., & Grant, M. (2015). *The Routledge handbook of planning for health and well-being: Shaping a sustainable and healthy future.* Routledge.

© The Editor(s) (if applicable) and The Author(s), under exclusive license to Springer Nature Switzerland AG 2022
P. Harris, *Illuminating Policy for Health*, Palgrave Studies in Public Health Policy Research,
https://doi.org/10.1007/978-3-031-13199-8

Baum, F., Delany-Crowe, T., Fisher, M., MacDougall, C., Harris, P., McDermott, D., & Marinova, D. (2018). Qualitative protocol for understanding the contribution of Australian policy in the urban planning, justice, energy and environment sectors to promoting health and health equity. *BMJ Open, 8*(9).

Baumgartner, F. R., Jones, B. D., & Mortensen, P. B. (2014). Punctuated equilibrium theory: Explaining stability and change in public policymaking. In C. Weible, & P. Sabatier (Eds), *Theories of the policy process* (pp. 59–103).

Bennett, R. G. (2000). Coastal planning on the Atlantic fringe, north Norway: The power game. *Ocean & Coastal Management, 43*(10–11), 879–904.

Bhaskar, R. (1978). *A realist theory of science* (3rd ed.). Verso.

Bilodeau, A., & Potvin, L. (2018). Unpacking complexity in public health interventions with the actor-network theory. *Health Promotion International, 33*(1), 173–181.

Bradford, N. J. (2005). *Place-based public policy: Towards a new urban and community agenda for Canada.* Canadian Policy Research Networks, Work Network.

Brandtner, C., Höllerer, M. A., Meyer, R. E., & Kornberger, M. (2017). Enacting governance through strategy: A comparative study of governance configurations in Sydney and Vienna. *Urban Studies, 54*(5), 1075–1091.

Brenner, N. (2009). What is critical urban theory? *City, 13*(2–3), 198–207.

Brenner, N. (2019). *New urban spaces: Urban theory and the scale question.* Oxford University Press.

Cairney, P. (2011). *Understanding public policy: Theories and issues.* Palgrave Macmillan.

Cairney, P. (2013). Standing on the shoulders of giants: How do we combine the insights of multiple theories in public policy studies? *Policy Studies Journal, 41*(1), 1–21.

Cairney, P., Heikkila, T., & Wood, M. (2019). *Making policy in a complex world.* Cambridge University Press.

Cairney, P., St Denny, E., & Mitchell, H. (2021). The future of public health policymaking after COVID-19: A qualitative systematic review of lessons from Health in All Policies. *Open Research Europe, 1*, 23.

Carstensen, M. B., & Schmidt, V. A. (2016). Power through, over and in ideas: Conceptualizing ideational power in discursive institutionalism. *Journal of European Public Policy, 23*(3), 318–337.

Cashmore, M., & Kornov, L. (2013). Changing theory of impact assessment. In A. Bond & R. Howitt (Eds.), *Sustainability appraisal: Pluralism, practice and progress. Natural and Built Environment Series* (pp. 18–33). Routledge.

Cashmore, M., Richardson, T., Hilding-Ryedvik, T., & Emmelin, L. (2010). Evaluating the effectiveness of impact assessment instruments: Theorising the nature and implications of their political constitution. *Environmental Impact Assessment Review, 30*(6), 371–379.

Clarke, S. E. (2015). Emerging research agendas. In K. Mossberger, S. E. Clarke, & P. John (Eds.), *The Oxford handbook of urban politics*.

Clegg, S. R. (1989). *Frameworks of power*. Sage.

Collier, A. (1994). *An Introduction to Roy Bhaskar's Philosophy*. Verso.

Commonwealth of Australia. (2016). Australian transport assessment and planning guidelines. Department of Infrastructure, Transport, Regional Development, Communication and the Arts. Canberra, Australia.

Connolly, J., Pyper, R., & van der Zwet, A. (2021). Governing 'levelling-up' in the UK: challenges and prospects. *Contemporary Social Science, 16*(5), 1–15.

Corburn, J. (2009). *Toward the healthy city: people, places, and the politics of urban planning*. Mit Press.

Corburn, J. (2017a). *Equitable and healthy city planning: Towards healthy urban governance in the century of the city* (pp. 31–41). Springer.

Corburn, J. (2017b). Urban place and health equity: Critical issues and practices. *International Journal of Environmental Research and Public Health, 14*(2), 117.

Cox, L. (2021, February 17). 'Development should stop': serious flaws in offsets plan for new western Sydney airport. *The Guardian*.

Cresswell, T. (2014). *Place: An introduction*. Wiley.

Crotty, M. (1998). *The foundations of social research: Meaning and perspective in the research process*. Sage.

Cummins, S., Curtis, S., Diez-Roux, A. V., & Macintyre, S. (2007). Understanding and representing 'place' in health research: A relational approach. *Social Science & Medicine, 65*(9), 1825–1838.

Dahlgren, G., & Whitehead, M. (1991). *Policies and strategies to promote social equity in health*. Stockholm: Institute for Future Studies.

Danermark, B., Ekstrom, L., Jakobsen, L., & Karlsson, J. C. (2002). *Explaining society: Critical realism and the social sciences*. Routledge.

Davies, J. S., & Imbroscio, D. L. (2009). *Theories of urban politics*. Sage.

Davies, J. S., & J. Trounstine (2012a). Urban politics and the new institutionalism. In K. Mossberger, S. E. Clarke, & P. John (Eds.), *The Oxford handbook of urban politics* (pp. 51–70).

Davies, J. S., & Trounstine, J. (2012b). Urban politics and the new institutionalism. In K. Mossberger, S. E. Clarke, & P. John (Eds.), *The Oxford handbook of new urban politics*.

De Leeuw, E. (2009). Evidence for healthy cities: Reflections on practice, method and theory. *Health Promotion International, 24*(suppl_1): i19-i36.

De Leeuw, E. (2012). Do healthy cities work? A logic of method for assessing impact and outcome of healthy cities. *Journal of Urban Health, 89*(2), 217–231.

de Leeuw, E. (2017a). *Cities and health from the neolithic to the anthropocene* (pp. 3–30). Springer.

De Leeuw, E. (2017b). Engagement of sectors other than health in integrated health governance, policy, and action. *Annual Review of Public Health, 38*(1), 329–349.

De Leeuw, E., & Harris, P. (2022). Governance and policies for setings based work. In S. Kokko (Ed.), *Handbook of settings based health promotion.* Springer Nature.

de Leeuw, E., Harris, P., Kim, J., & Yashadhana, A. (2021, December). A health political science for health promotion. *Global Health Promotion, 28*(4), 17–25.

de Leeuw, E., & Skovgaard, T. (2005). Utility-driven evidence for healthy cities: Problems with evidence generation and application. *Social Science & Medicine, 61*(6), 1331–1341.

Downward, P., Finch, J. H., & Ramsay, J. (2002). Critical realism, empirical methods and inference: A critical discussion. *Cambridge Journal of Economics, 26*(4), 481–500.

Elling, B. (2009). Rationality and effectiveness: Does EIA/SEA treat them as synonyms? *Impact Assessment and Project Appraisal, 27*(2), 121–131.

Fafard, P. (2015). Beyond the usual suspects: Using political science to enhance public health policy making. *JECH, 69*(11), 1129–1132.

Fafard, P., Cassola, A., & de Leeuw, E. (2021). *Public health political science: Integrating science and politics for public health.* Springer.

Fairclough, N. (2003). *Analysing discourse: Textual analysis for social research.* Psychology Press.

Fincher, R., Pardy, M., & Shaw, K. (2016). Place-making or place-masking? The everyday political economy of "making place." *Planning Theory and Practice, 17*(4), 516–536.

Flyvbjerg, B. (1998). *Rationality and power: Democracy in practice.* University of Chicago Press.

Flyvbjerg, B. (2001). *Making social science matter: Why social inquiry fails and how it can succeed again.* Cambridge University Press.

Flyvbjerg, B., Bruzelius, N., & Rothengatter, W. (2003). *Megaprojects and risk: An anatomy of ambition.* Cambridge University Press.

Fonseca, M. (2016). *Gramsci's critique of civil society: Towards a new concept of hegemony.* Routledge.

Friel, S., Harris, P., Simpson, S., Bhushan, A., & Baer, B. (2015). Health in all policies approaches: Pearls from the Western Pacific Region. *Asia & the Pacific Policy Studies, 2*(2), 324–337.

Friel, S., Townsend, B., Fisher, M., Harris, P., Freeman, T., & Baum, F. J. (2021, August). Power and the people's health. *Social Science and Medicine, 282,* 114173.

Fuchs, D., & Lederer, M. M. (2007). The power of business. *Business and Politics, 9*(3), 1–17.

Garcia, M., & Judd, D. R. (2012). Competitive cities. In K. Mossberger, S. E. Clarke, & P. John (Eds.), *The Oxford handbook of urban politics.*

Gaventa, J. (2006). Finding the spaces for change: A power analysis. *IDS Bulletin, 37*(6), 23–33.

Giles-Corti, B., Vernez-Moudon, A., Reis, R., Turrell, G., Dannenberg, A. L., Badland, H., Foster, S., Lowe, M., Sallis, J. F., & Stevenson, M. (2016). City planning and population health: A global challenge. *The Lancet, 388*(10062), 2912–2924.

Gillen, M. (2004). Promoting place: Elevating place-based discourse and new approaches in local governance in New South Wales. *Urban Policy and Research, 22*(2), 207–220.

Glaser, B., & Strauss, A. (1967). *The discovery of grounded theory.* Aldine.

Greiss, G., & Piracha, A. (2021). Post-political planning in Sydney: A turn in the wrong direction. *Australian Planner, 57*, 1–10.

Haigh, F., Fletcher-Lartey, S., Jaques, K., Millen, E., Calalang, C., de Leeuw, E., Mahimbo, A., & Hirono, K. (2020). The health impacts of transformative infrastructure change: Process matters as much as outcomes. *Environmental Impact Assessment Review, 85*, 106437.

Hall, P. A., & Taylor, R. C. R. (1996). Political Science and the Three New Institutionalisms. *Political Studies, 44*(5), 936.

Hamlin, C., & Sidley, P. (1998). Revolutions in public health: 1848, and 1998? *BMJ, 317*(7158), 587.

Hancock, T. (1985). Beyond health care: From public health policy to healthy public policy. *Canadian Journal of Public Health, 76*(Suppl 1), 9–11.

Harris, P., Baum, F., Friel, S., Mackean, T., Schram, A., & Townsend, B. (2020a). A glossary of theories for understanding power and policy for health equity. *Journal of Epidemiology and Community Health, 74*, 548–552.

Harris, P., Baum, F., Friel, S., Mackean, T., Schram, A., & Townsend, B. (2020b). A glossary of theories for understanding power and policy for health equity. *Journal of Epidemiology and Community Health, 74*(6), 548–552.

Harris, P., Riley, E., Sainsbury, P., Kent, J., Baum, F., & Lane, A. (2016a). *Assessing environmental impacts of major transport infrastructure projects: Where does human health fit?* University of Sydney.

Harris, P., Fisher, M., Friel, S., Sainsbury, P., Harris, E., De Leeuw, E., & Baum, F. (2022). City deals and health equity in Sydney Australia. *Health & Place, 73.* https://doi.org/10.1016/j.healthplace.2021.102711

Harris, P., Friel, S., & Wilson, A. (2015a). 'Including health in systems responsible for urban planning': A realist policy analysis research programme. *British Medical Journal Open, 5*(7), e008822.

Harris, P., & Haigh, F. (2015). Including health in environmental impact assessments: Is an institutional approach useful for practice? *Impact Assessment and Project Appraisal, 33*(2), 135–141.

Harris, P., Haigh, F., Thornell, M., Molloy, L., & Sainsbury, P. (2014a). Housing, health and master planning: Rules of engagement. *Public Health, 128*(4), 354–359.

Harris, P., Kent, J., Sainsbury, P., Marie-Thow, A., Baum, F., Friel, S., & McCue, P. (2018a). Creating 'healthy built environment' legislation in Australia; A policy analysis. *Health Promotion International, 33*(6), 1090–1100.

Harris, P., Kent, J., Sainsbury, P., Riley, E., Sharma, N., & Harris, E. (2020c). Healthy urban planning: an institutional policy analysis of strategic planning in Sydney, Australia. *Health Promotion International, 35*(5), 1251.

Harris, P., Kent, J., Sainsbury, P., & Thow, A.-M. (2016b). Framing health for land-use planning legislation: A qualitative descriptive content analysis. *Social Science & Medicine, 148*, 42–51.

Harris, P., McManus, P., Sainsbury, P., Viliani, F., & Riley, E. (2021). The institutional dynamics behind limited human health considerations in environmental assessments of coal mining projects in New South Wales, Australia. *Environmental Impact Assessment Review, 86*, 106473.

Harris, P., Riley, E., Dawson, A., Friel, S., & Lawson, K. (2020d). "Stop talking around projects and talk about solutions": Positioning health within infrastructure policy to achieve the sustainable development goals. *Health Policy, 124*(6), 591–598.

Harris, P., Riley, E., Sainsbury, P., Kent, J., & Baum, F. (2018b). Including health in environmental impact assessments of three mega transport projects in Sydney, Australia: A critical, institutional, analysis. *Environmental Impact Assessment Review, 68*, 109–116.

Harris, P., Sainsbury, P., & Kemp, L. (2014b). The fit between health impact assessment and public policy: Practice meets theory. *Social Science & Medicine, 108*, 46–53.

Harris, P., Viliani, F., & Spickett, J. (2015b). Assessing health impacts within environmental impact assessments: An opportunity for public health globally which must not remain missed. *International Journal of Environmental Research and Public Health, 12*(1), 1044–1049.

Harris, P., & Wise, M. (2020). *Healthy public policy.* Oxford University Press.

Harris, P. J., Harris-Roxas, B. F., & Harris, E. (2007). An overview of the regulatory planning system in New South Wales: Identifying points of intervention for health impact assessment and consideration of health impacts. *New South Wales Public Health Bulletin, 18*(10), 188–191.

Harris, P. J., Kemp, L. A., & Sainsbury, P. (2012). The essential elements of health impact assessment and healthy public policy: A qualitative study of practitioner perspectives. *British Medical Journal Open, 2*(6), e001245.

Harvey, D. (1987). Reconsidering social theory: A debate. *Environment and Planning d: Society and Space, 5*(4), 367–434.

Harvey, D. (1989). From managerialism to entrepreneurialism: The transformation in urban governance in late capitalism. *Geografiska Annaler: Series b, Human Geography, 71*(1), 3–17.

Harvey, D. (2001). *Spaces of capital: Towards a critical geography.* Routledge.

Haugaard, M. (2003). Reflections on seven ways of creating power. *European Journal of Social Theory, 6*(1), 87–113.

Haughton, G., & McManus, P. (2019). Participation in postpolitical times. *Journal of the American Planning Association, 85*(3), 321–334.

Healey, P. (2006a). Transforming governance: Challenges of institutional adaptation and a new politics of space. *European Planning Studies, 14*(3), 299–320.

Healey, P. (2006b). *Urban complexity and spatial strategies: Towards a relational planning for our times.* Routledge.

Healey, P., Cars, G., Madanipour, A., & De Magalhaes, C. (2002a). Transforming governance, institutionalist analysis and institutional capacity. In G. Cars, P. Healey, A. Madanipour, & C. De Magalhães (Eds.), *Urban governance, institutional capacity and social milieux* (pp. 20–42). Routledge.

Healey, P., Cars, G., Madanipour, A., & de Magalhães, C. (2002b). Urban governance capacity in complex societies: challenges of institutional adaptation. In G. Cars, P. Healey, A., Madanipour, & C. De Magalhães (Eds.), *Urban governance, institutional capacity and social milieux* (pp. 204–225).

Heikkila, T., & Cairney, P. (2018). *Comparison of theories of the policy process* (pp. 301–327). Routledge.

Hooper, P., Foster, S., Bull, F., Knuiman, M., Christian, H., Timperio, A., Wood, L., Trapp, G., Boruff, B., & Francis, J. J. (2020). Living liveable? RESIDE's evaluation of the "Liveable Neighborhoods" planning policy on the health supportive behaviors and wellbeing of residents in Perth, Western Australia. *Social Science and Medicine Population Health, 10,* 100538.

Horton, R. (2017). Offline: Medicine and Marx *Lancet 390,* 20126.

Howarth, D. (2010). Power, discourse, and policy: Articulating a hegemony approach to critical policy studies. *Critical Policy Studies, 3*(3–4), 309–335.

Howlett, M., Ramesh, M., & Perl, A. (2009). *Studying public policy: Policy cycles and policy sub-systems* (3rd ed.). Oxford University Press.

Hresc, J., Riley, E., & Harris, P. (2018). Mining project's economic impact on local communities, as a social determinant of health: A documentary analysis of environmental impact statements. *Environmental Impact Assessment Review, 72,* 64–70.

Hu, R. (2019). City deals: Old wine in new bottles? In M. Evans, M. Grattan, & B. McCaffrie (Eds.), *From turnbull to morrison: Understanding the trust divide.* Melbourne University Press.

Immergut, E. M. (1998). The theoretical core of the new institutionalism. *Politics & Society, 26*(1), 5–34.

Immergut, E. M. (2006). *Historical-institutionalism in political science and the problem of change* (pp. 237–259). Springer.

Jenkins-Smith, H., Nohrstedt, D., Weible, C., & Sabatier, P. (2014). The advocacy coalition framework: Foundations, evolution, and ongoing research. In P. Sabatier & C. Weible (Eds.), *Theories of the policy process*. Routledge.

Jessop, B. (1998). The rise of governance and the risks of failure: The case of economic development. *International Social Science Journal, 50*(155), 29–45.

Jessop, B. (2001). Institutional re(turns) and the strategic—Relational approach. *33*(7): 1213–1235.

Jessop, B. (2002). Liberalism, neoliberalism, and urban governance: A state–theoretical perspective. *Antipode, 34*(3), 452–472.

Jessop, B. (2005). Critical realism and the strategic-relational approach. *New Formations, 56*(1), 40–53.

Jessop, B. (2007). *State power*. Polity.

John, P. (2003). Is there life after policy streams, advocacy coalitions, and punctuations: Using evolutionary theory to explain policy change? *Policy Studies Journal, 31*(4), 481–498.

Jonas, A. E., & Ward, K. (2007). Introduction to a debate on city-regions: New geographies of governance, democracy and social reproduction. *International Journal of Urban and Regional Research, 31*(1), 169–178.

Jones, B. D. (1994). *Reconceiving decision-making in democratic politics: Attention, choice, and public policy*. University of Chicago Press.

Jones, B. D., & Baumgartner, F. R. (2012). From there to here: Punctuated equilibrium to the general punctuation thesis to a theory of government information processing. *Policy Studies Journal, 40*(1), 1–20.

Jordan, D. P. (1995). *Transforming Paris: The life and labors of Baron Haussman*. Simon and Schuster.

Kay, A. (2005). A critique of the use of path dependency in policy studies. *Public Administration, 83*(3), 553–571.

Kent, J. L., Harris, P., Sainsbury, P., Baum, F., McCue, P., & Thompson, S. (2018). Influencing urban planning policy: An exploration from the perspective of public health. *Urban Policy and Research, 36*(1), 20–34.

Kincheloe, J. L. (2011). On to the next level: Continuing the conceptualization of the bricolage. *Key works in critical pedagogy* (pp. 253–277). Brill.

Kingdon, J. W. (2011). *Agendas, alternatives, and public policies* (3rd ed.). Ill, Pearson Education Inc.

Kjær, A. M. (2009). Governance and the urban bureaucracy. In J. S. Davies & D. L. Imbroscio (Eds.), *Theories of urban politics* (pp. 137–152). Sage.

Koch, P. (2013). Overestimating the shift from government to governance: Evidence from Swiss metropolitan areas. *Governance, 26*(3), 397–423.

Larsen, K. (2007). *The health impacts of place-based interventions in areas of concentrated disadvantaged: A review of literature*. Sydney South West Area Health Service, NSW Health.

Laumann, E. O., & Knoke, D. (1987). *The organizational state: Social choice in national policy domains*. University of Wisconsin Press.

Lawless, A. P., Baum, F., Delany, T., MacDougall, C. J., Williams, C., McDermott, D. R., & van Eyk, H. C. (2017). Developing a framework for a program theory-based approach to evaluating policy processes and outcomes: Health in all policies in South Australia. *International Journal of Health Policy and Management, 7*(6), 510–521.

Lawson, T. (2003). *Reorienting economics*. Routledge.

Layder, D. (1998). *Sociological practice: Linking theory and social research*. Sage.

Litman, T. (2013). Transportation and public health. *Annual Review of Public Health, 34*, 217–233.

Lowndes, V. (2001). Rescuing Aunt Sally: Taking institutional theory seriously in urban politics. *Urban Studies, 38*(11), 1953–1971.

Lowndes, V. (2009). New institutionalism and urban politics. *Theories of Urban Politics, 2*, 91–105.

Lukes, S. (2005). *Power: A radical view*. Palgrave Macmillan.

Macintyre, S., Ellaway, A., & Cummins, S. (2002). Place effects on health: How can we conceptualise, operationalise and measure them? *Social Science & Medicine, 55*(1), 125–139.

Marsh, D. (2009). Keeping ideas in their place: In praise of thin constructivism. *Australian Journal of Political Science, 44*(4), 679–696.

McCann, E. (2017). Governing urbanism: Urban governance studies 1.0, 2.0 and beyond. *Urban Studies, 54*(2), 312–326.

McGowan, V. J., Buckner, S., Mead, R., McGill, E., Ronzi, S., Beyer, F., & Bambra, C. (2021). Examining the effectiveness of place-based interventions to improve public health and reduce health inequalities: An umbrella review. *BMC Public Health, 21*(1), 1–17.

McGreevy, M., Harris, P., Delaney-Crowe, T., Fisher, M., Sainsbury, P., & Baum, F. (2020a). The power of collaborative planning: How a health and planning collaboration facilitated integration of health goals in the 30-year plan for Greater Adelaide. *Urban Policy and Research, 38*(3), 262–275.

McGreevy, M., Harris, P., Delaney-Crowe, T., Fisher, M., Sainsbury, P., Riley, E., & Baum, F. (2020b). How well do Australian government urban planning policies respond to the social determinants of health and health equity? *J Land Use Policy, 99*, 105053.

McGreevy, M., Harris, P., Delany-Crowe, T., Fisher, M., Sainsbury, P., & Baum, F. (2019). Can health and health equity be advanced by urban planning strategies designed to advance global competitiveness? Lessons from two Australian case studies. *Social Science & Medicine, 242*, 112594.

McGuirk, P. (2005). Neoliberalist planning? Re-thinking and re-casting Sydney's metropolitan planning. *Geographical Research, 43*(1), 59–70.

McGuirk, P. (2007). The political construction of the city-region: Notes from Sydney. *International Journal of Urban and Regional Research, 31*(1), 179–187.

McManus, P. (2022). Infrastructure, health and urban planning: Rethinking the past and exploring future possibilities. *Infrastructure and Health* (In press).

McManus, P., & Haughton, G. (2021). Fighting to undo a deal: Identifying and resisting the financialization of the WestConnex motorway, Sydney, Australia. *Environment Planning a: Economy Space, 53*(1), 131–149.

McQueen, D. and L. M. Anderson (2001). What counts as evidence: issues and debates. In I. Rootman, M. Goodstadt, B. Hyndman, D. V. McQueen, L. Potvin, J. Springett, & E. Ziglio et al. (Eds.), *Evaluation in Health Promotion. Principles and Perspectives.* (pp. 63–82). WHO Regional Publications, Copenhagen. European Series: 63–81.

Medvetz, T., & Sallaz, J. J. (2018). *The Oxford handbook of Pierre Bourdieu.* Oxford University Press.

Merton, R. (1967). *On theoretical sociology.* Free Press.

Milio, N. (1981). *Promoting health through public policy.* Davis.

Milio, N. (1987). Making healthy public policy; developing the science by learning the art: An ecological framework for policy studies. *Health Promotion International, 2*(3), 263–274.

Milio, N. (2001). Glossary: Healthy public policy. *Journal of Epidemiology & Community Health, 55*(9), 622–623.

Mingers, J. (2014). *Systems thinking, critical realism and philosophy: A confluence of ideas.* Routledge.

Morgan, R. K. (2012). Environmental impact assessment: The state of the art. *Impact Assessment and Project Appraisal, 30*(1), 5–14.

Morrison, N., & Van Den Nouwelant, R. (2020). Western Sydney's urban transformation: Examining the governance arrangements driving forward the growth vision. *J Australian Planner, 56*(2), 73–82.

Mossberger, K. (2009). Urban regime analysis. *Theories of urban politics, 2*, 40–54.

Mossberger, K., Clarke, S. E., & John, P. (2015). *The Oxford handbook of urban politics.* Oxford University Press.

Mossberger, K., & Stoker, G. (2001). The evolution of urban regime theory: The challenge of conceptualization. *Urban Affairs Review, 36*(6), 810–835.

Navarro, V. (2009). What we mean by social determinants of health. *J International Journal of Health Services, 39*(3), 423–441.

Neveu, E. (2018). Bourdieu's capital(s): Sociologizing an economic concept. In T. Medvetz & J. J. Sallaz (Eds.), *The Oxford Handbook of Pierre Bourdieu.*

NSW Government. (2015). Greater Sydney Commission Act 2015 No 57. NSW Legislation. NSW Government.

NSW Government. (2021a). Infrastructure procurement framework. Infrastructure NSW. NSW Government.

NSW Government. (2021b). New community commissioner for aerotropolis: Ministerial media release: NSW Department of Planning and Environment. NSW Government.

NSW Government Office of the Government Architect. (2018). *Better placed*, from https://www.governmentarchitect.nsw.gov.au/policies/better-placed.

NSW Legislation. (2019). Environmental planning and assessment act 1979 No 203. https://www.legislation.nsw.gov.au/#/view/act/1979/203.

NSW Treasury Department. (2021). *FMT reforms*, from https://www.treasury.nsw.gov.au/budget-financial-management/reform.

Ollman, B. (2001). Critical realism in the light of Marx's process of abstraction. In J. Lopez & G. Potter (Eds.), *After postmodernism: An introduction to critical realism.*

Outhwaite, W. (1987). *New philosophies of social science: Realism, hermeneutics and critical theory.* MacMillan.

Painter, M. (2001). Multi-level governance and the emergence of collaborative federal institutions in Australia. *Policy & Politics, 29*(2), 137–150.

Pawson, R. (1996). Theorizing the interview. *British Journal of Sociology, 47*, 295–314.

Pawson, R. (2013). *The science of evaluation: A realist manifesto.* Sage.

Pawson, R., & Tilley, N. (1997). *Realistic evaluation.* Sage.

Peters, B. G. (2019). *Institutional theory in political science: The new institutionalism.* Edward Elgar Publishing.

Petticrew, M., Tugwell, P., Welch, V., Ueffing, E., Kristjansson, E., Armstrong, R., Doyle, J., & Waters, E. (2009). Better evidence about wicked issues in tackling health inequities. *Journal of Public Health, 31*(3), 453–456.

Pickett, K., & Wilkinson, R. (2010). *The spirit level: Why equality is better for everyone.* Penguin UK.

Pierre, J. (1999a). Models of Urban Governance: The institutional dimension of urban politics. *Urban Affairs Review, 34*(3), 372–396.

Pierre, J. (1999b). Models of urban governance: The institutional dimension of urban politics. *J Urban Affairs Review, 34*(3), 372–396.

Pierre, J. (2011). *The politics of urban governance.* Palgrave Macmillan.

Pierre, J., & Peters, B. G. (2012). Urban governance. In K. Mossberger, S. E. Clarke, & P. John (Eds.), *The Oxford handbook of urban politics.*

Pill, M. (2021). *Governing cities: Politics and policy.* Springer.

Potter, G., & Lopez, P. (2001). After postmodernism: The new millennium. In J. Lopez & G. Potter (Eds.), *After postmodernism: An introduction to critical realism.*

PPS. (2016). *Placemaking—what if we built our cities around places?* Project for Public Places.

Pratt, A. C. (1995). Putting critical realism to work: The practical implications for geographical research. *Progress in Human Geography, 19*(1), 61–74.

QSR International Pty Ltd. NVivo. https://www.qsrinternational.com/nvivo-qualitative-data-analysis-software/home, QSR International.

Raphael, D. (2014). Beyond policy analysis: The raw politics behind opposition to healthy public policy. *Health Promotion International, 30*(2), 380–396.

Real-Dato, J. (2009). Mechanisms of policy change: A proposal for a synthetic explanatory framework. *Journal of Comparative Policy Analysis: Research and Practice, 11*(1), 117–143.

Rein, M., & Schön, D. (1994). *Frame reflection: Toward the resolution of intractable policy controversies.* Basic Book.

Rein, M., & Schön, D. (1996). Frame-critical policy analysis and frame-reflective policy practice. *Knowledge and Policy, 9*(1), 85–104.

Rhodes, R. A. (2007). Understanding governance: Ten years on. *Organization Studies, 28*(8), 1243–1264.

Richardson, T. (2005). Environmental assessment and planning theory: Four short stories about power, multiple rationality, and ethics. *Environmental Impact Assessment Review, 25*(4), 341–365.

Riley, E., Harris, P., Kent, J., Sainsbury, P., Lane, A., & Baum, F. (2017). Including health in environmental assessments of major transport infrastructure projects: A documentary analysis. *International Journal of Health Policy and Management, 7*(2), 144–153.

Riley, E., Sainsbury, P., McManus, P., Colagiuri, R., Viliani, F., Dawson, A., Duncan, E., Stone, Y., Pham, T., & Harris, P. (2019). Including health impacts in environmental impact assessments for three Australian coal-mining projects: A documentary analysis. *Health Promotion International, 35*(3), 449–457.

Robertson, T., McCarthy, A., Jegasothy, E., & Harris, P. (2021a). Urban transport infrastructure planning and the public interest: A public health perspective. *Public Health Research and Practice, 31*(2), 3122108.

Robertson, T. J., McCarthy, A., Jegasothy, E., & Harris, P. (2021b). Urban transport infrastructure planning and the public interest: a public health perspective. *31*(2), e3122108

Rode, P. (2019). Urban planning and transport policy integration: The role of governance hierarchies and networks in London and Berlin. *Journal of Urban Affairs, 41*(1), 39–63.

Rubin, H. J., & Rubin, I. S. (2011). *Qualitative interviewing: The art of hearing data.* Sage.

Rushton, C. (2014). Whose place is it anyway? Representational politics in a place-based health initiative. *Health & Place, 26*, 100–109.

Sabatier, P. A. (1988). An advocacy coalition framework of policy change and the role of policy-oriented learning therein. *Policy Sciences, 21*(2), 129–168.

Sabatier, P. A. (1998). The advocacy coalition framework: Revisions and relevance for Europe. *Journal of European Public Policy, 5*(1), 98–130.

Sabatier, P. A., & Weible, C. (2014). *Theories of the policy process*. Westview Press.

Sapotichne, J., & Jones, B. D. (2012). *Setting city agendas: Power and policy change*. Oxford University Press.

Savage, V., & Yeh, P. (2019). Novelist Cormac McCarthy's tips on how to write a great science paper. *Nature, 574*(7778), 441.

Sayer, A. (1992). *Method in social science: A realist approach* (2nd ed.). Routledge.

Sayer, A. (1998). Abstraction: A realist interpretation. In M. Archer, R. Bhaskar, A. Collier, T. Lawson, & A. Norrie (Eds.), *Critical realism: Essential readings* (pp. 120–143). Routledge.

Sayer, A. (2000). *Realism and social science*. Sage.

Schaler, E. (2014). An assessment of the institutional analysis and development framework and introduction of the social-ecological systems framework. In P. Sabatier & C. Weible (Eds.), *Theories of the Policy Process* (p. 267). Westview.

Schmidt, V. A. (2008). Discursive institutionalism: The explanatory power of ideas and discourse. *Annual Review of Political Science, 11*, 303–326.

Schultz, M. (2008). Rudolf Virchow. *Emerging Infectious Diseases, 14*(9), 1480.

Schwarzman, J., Bauman, A., Gabbe, B. J., Rissel, C., Shilton, T., Smith, B. J. J. E., & Planning, P. (2021). How practitioner, organisational and system-level factors act to influence health promotion evaluation capacity: Validation of a conceptual framework. *Evaluation and Program Planning, 91*, 102019.

Scott, A. J., & Storper, M. (2015). The nature of cities: The scope and limits of urban theory. *International Journal of Urban and Regional Research, 39*(1), 1–15.

Scott, W. R. (2005). *Institutions and Organizations: Ideas and Interests* (3rd ed.). Sage Publications.

Searle, G., & Legacy, C. (2021). Locating the public interest in mega infrastructure planning: The case of Sydney's WestConnex. *Urban Studies, 58*(4), 826–844.

Smith, K. (2013). *Beyond evidence based policy in public health: The interplay of ideas*. Springer.

Smith, K. E. (2006). Problematising power relations in 'elite' interviews. *Geoforum, 37*(4), 643–653.

Smith, K. E., & Katikireddi, S. V. (2013). A glossary of theories for understanding policymaking. *Journal of Epidemiology and Community Health, 67*(2), 198–202.

Steele, W. (2011). Strategy-making for sustainability: An institutional learning approach to transformative planning practice. *Planning Theory & Practice, 12*(2), 205–221.

Stoker, G. (1998). Governance as theory: Five propositions. *International Social Science Journal, 50*(155), 17–28.

Stone, C. N. (2005). Looking back to look forward: Reflections on urban regime analysis. *Urban Affairs Review, 40*(3), 309–341.

Stone, C. N. (2015). Power. In E. Mossberger, S. Clarke, & J. Peter (Eds.), *Oxford handbook of urban politics.* Oxford University Press.

Stone, D. A. (1997). *Policy paradox: The art of political decision making.* Norton New York.

Stones, R. (1996). *Sociological reasoning: Towards a past-modern sociology.* Macmillan Press.

Swyngedouw, E. (2005). Governance innovation and the citizen: The Janus face of governance-beyond-the-state. *Urban Studies, 42*(11), 1991–2006.

Swyngedouw, E. (2009). The antinomies of the postpolitical city. In search of a democratic politics of environmental production. *International Journal of Urban and Regional Research, 33*(3), 601–620.

Szreter, S. (2005). *Health and wealth Studies in history and policy.* Boydell and Brewer.

Szreter, S., Kinmonth, A. L., Kriznik, N. M., & Kelly, M. P. (2016). Health, welfare, and the state—The dangers of forgetting history. *The Lancet, 388*(10061), 2734–2735.

Tesh, S., Tuohy, C., Christoffel, T., Hancock, T., Norsigian, J., Nightingale, E., & Robertson, L. (1987). The meaning of healthy public policy. *Health Promotion International, 2*(3), 257–262.

van der Heijden, J., J. Kuhlmann, Lindquist, E., & Wellstead, A. (2019). Have policy process scholars embraced causal mechanisms? A review of five popular frameworks. *Public Policy and Administration.* 0952076718814894.

Weible, C. M. (2014). Introducing the scope and focus of policy process research and theory. In P. W. Sabatier & M. Christopher (Eds.), *Theories of the policy process* (p. 1). Westview Press.

Weible, C. M., & Sabatier, P. (2018). *Theories of the policy process.* Routledge.

Weiss, C. H. (1999). The interface between evaluation and public policy. *Evaluation, 5*(4), 468–486.

Williams, S. J. (2003). Beyond meaning, discourse and the empirical world: Critical realist reflections on health. *Social Theory & Health, 1*, 42–71.

Winslow, C.-E. (1920). The untilled fields of public health. *Science, 51*, 23–33.

World Health Organisation. (2008). *Closing the gap in a generation: Health equity through action on the social determinants of health.* Final Report of the Commission on Social Determinants of Health. Geneva, World Health Organization.

World Health Organization. (1986). *Ottawa charter for health promotion.* Geneva.

Yeung, H. W. C. (1997). Critical realism and realist research in human geography: A method or a philosophy in search of a method? *Progress in Human Geography, 21*(1), 51–74.

Yin, R. K. (2012). *Case study research: Design and methods.* Sage.

Zahariadis, N. (2014). Ambiguity and multiple streams. In P. Sabatier & C. Weible (Eds.), *Theories of the policy process* (pp. 25–58). Westview Press.

INDEX